4⁰⁰

> **BEES DON'T GET ARTHRITIS** <

> > IMPORTANT NOTICE < <

> Some people are violently allergic to <
bee stings, often without their knowl-
> edge, and if stung can have a severe, <
perhaps fatal reaction.
>
It is vital that before beginning any <
program of bee venom therapy the
> reader get a doctor to test him or her <
> for this allergy. <

BEES DON'T GET ARTHRITIS

ARTHRITIS

Fred Malone

Thomas Congdon Books

E.P. DUTTON · NEW YORK

Copyright © 1979 by Fred Malone

All rights reserved. Printed in the U.S.A.

For information contact:
E.P. Dutton, 2 Park Avenue, New York, N.Y. 10016

Library of Congress Cataloging in Publication Data

Malone, Fred.
  Bees don't get arthritis.

  "Thomas Congdon books."
  Bibliography: p.
1.–Bee venom—Therapeutic use. 2.–Arthritis. 3.–Bee products—Therapeutic use. 4.–Arthritis—Bibliography. 5.–Malone, Fred. I.–Title.
RM666.B38M34   616.7'2   78–17066

ISBN:0-525-06240-8

Published simultaneously in Canada by Clarke, Irwin & Company Limited, Toronto and Vancouver

10 9 8 7 6 5 4 3 2

TO
My lady, Jeannie

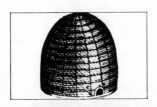

INTRODUCTION

by George Vogel, M.D., D.A.B.F.P., P.C.

SIR WILLIAM OSLER once said, "Humanity has but three great enemies: fever, famine and war. Of these by far the greatest, by far the most terrible, is fever." In the century since Osler made this observation, though famine and war have persisted, fever has been conquered. Today, however, Osler would most likely add arthritis to the enemy list. This disease has plagued mankind from the beginning, but only in recent years have we come to understand just how widespread and costly this illness is. As a family practitioner, I have been keenly aware of the massive suffering caused by arthritis, but was not really until my dear wife was afflicted by a rapidly destructive and debilitating arthritis of the hips, resistant to all medical management and resulting in total hip replacements, could I fully appreciate the extent of the physical and emotional stress resulting from this enemy.

Some months ago, in his extraordinary pilgrimage around the country in search of information he hoped would bring understanding of arthritis, Fred Malone visited us at our home. He intrigued us with the story of the way bee venom had apparently alleviated the arthritis of his knees. We listened with fascination as he told of the research that has been done, in both the recent and distant past, on the effect of bee venom on arthritis and other human illnesses. It was of great interest to me that scientific work had been done in Russia and Germany and in prestigious scientific institutions in the United States. It is striking to note that investigators have already discovered a great deal about the way bee venom works in the human body, triggering complex immunological activities, and that the danger of overreaction to venom, such as anaphylactic shock, can be avoided thanks to the present understanding of these immunological responses.

Yet in spite of this work—by beekeepers, practicing physicians, and medical research centers—medical authorities have done little to promote the use of this knowledge. A potential source of relief to the multitudes of people suffering from arthritis has been denied them.

We in medicine have come up with remarkably few answers, and if others discover a promising treatment, I feel we are obliged to pursue it. Fred Malone's interesting book, with all its insights into the frustrations of humanity caused by unrelieved suffering, offers the possibility that man will accept help from non-medical sources. I hope the book will stimulate accelerated activity by medicine in this area.

Dr. Vogel has been a family practitioner for thirty-three years in Westchester County, New York, and has been Chief of Family Medicine at Phelps Memorial Hospital in North Tarrytown.

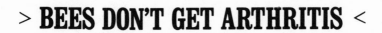

> **BEES DON'T GET ARTHRITIS** <

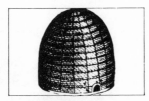

ONE

"DOCTOR, I'm coming down with a bad case of the blahs. You know, my stomach feels funny, my head is fixing to hurt. I've been around a lot of flu. Probably coming down with the flu."

"You're probably coming down with the flu."

"Well, now that I've got a second opinion, what are we going to do about it?"

"There's nothing we can do about flu. It's a virus, and we just don't know anything about it. Take some vitamins, get a lot of rest, and treat whatever local condition develops with your favorite remedy. Like aspirin for the headache, and so forth."

I went home and took vitamin C wildly, indiscriminately, by the handful. And I didn't get the flu. But—

"Doctor, I've had these sores from the base of my nose to the bottom of my throat for a week now and I'm going bananas."

"My God. I've never seen anything as bad as that. They must be cold sores or fever blisters, but I've never seen such a mess. That's awful."

"I know it's awful—that's why I'm here. What are we going to do about it?"

"Cold sores are caused by a virus just under the skin that

erupts occasionally. We don't know what to do about them. Just let them run their course and dry up."

A few weeks after the cold sores disappeared, I began to have a lot of pain in my knees. I had never had this trouble before and it worried me.

"Doctor, I can't have arthritis."

"Why not?"

"I'm too young."

"How old are you?"

"I was born two years before Amy Johnson flew solo from London to Australia in nineteen and a half days."

"Then you're about forty-seven. That's not too young."

"OK. I'm not too young. What are we going to do about it?"

"There's nothing we can do about arthritis except take aspirin and learn to live with it."

"Doctor, how are you boys on a compound fracture?"

"That we're good at."

"OK. I won't bother you again unless I break something, and at the rate I'm failing, I'll probably see you soon."

I lied. A week later the pain in my knees made me nauseous, and the aspirin wouldn't do a thing for me—so I went to my GP, who sent me to an orthopedic man. I had the usual gamut of blood tests and X rays. The results were negative, and in the absence of any other evidence or information the doctors concurred that I had arthritis. I was not examined for evidence of arthritis in any of my other joints, of which I have several.

And so the orthopedic man put me on Motrin, which is the same as aspirin and costs ten times as much.

Several months later, in the spring of the Bicentennial, I'm building a picket fence for Barry Nelson in Beverly Hills. I'm sort of down in the mouth because I'm thinking about these crazy knees and how they've screwed me up.

By even the most modest standards my physical components can be characterized as ordinary, and that's a generous appraisal. Except for my legs, which indeed were the marvel of the Western world. They were indefatigable machines, handsomely proportioned, keenly responsive to the most exacting demands. A joy and a comfort.

And now my sniveling kneeballs had seemingly destroyed a forty-seven-year tradition of leg yeomanry almost akin to greatness.

I took a lunch break and was sitting by the pool trying to tongue down a peanut butter sandwich when suddenly I had a flashback that was forcefully to alter the course of my life.

Perhaps it was the warm sunshine in my face, the moist fragrance of newly watered peat moss, maybe even the peanut butter, that produced the special alchemy.

It's 1962. I'm sitting by the fire munching a bit of Scotch with my new friend, Ray Murdoch. Strange and wondrous animal trophies hang on the wall in his Vermont home. Ray has regaled me with rich tales about Africa and India, given me a humorous and incisive minicourse in the snares of beef raising and a host of other subjects that marked him as a man of intelligence and genuine sophistication.

Then he got onto this business about gout.

"I had gout so badly in both thumbs that I couldn't get out of bed. The pain was so bad I dared not move. Doctors couldn't do a damn thing about it. I tell you, I couldn't get out of bed except with extreme discomfort.

"Well, after a couple of days of this, Gladys said why didn't I go over and see Charlie Mraz, the beekeeper."

"Beekeeper?" I said.

"Yes, beekeeper. Well, I figured what the hell—the doctors aren't doing anything for me. I might as well give Charlie a shot at it. So I went over and got a couple of bee stings in each thumb, and by morning the gout was gone and I've never been troubled again."

I smiled, for I had gone to college, read *Time* compulsively, and seen all the Dr. Kildare movies.

"Don't smile," Ray said. "There are hundreds of people in this area who have been cured of arthritis by Charlie and his bees."

Being in my prime (or so I thought), I completely dismissed the story from my mind. That is, until this day, when sun, moist peat moss (and maybe Kraft's peanut butter) summoned the conversation from my subconscious.

"Hot damn, Freddie boy—that's it! We're gonna get a few stings, drive that arthritis out, and restore these legs to near their former greatness," I said out loud.

We're gonna find Charlie Mraz in Vermont.

We're gonna go 25,000 miles down a lot of roads. We're gonna meet a bunch of really fine people. Best group of people we've ever met.

We're gonna be enraptured by honey and captivated by its goodness and mysteries.

We're gonna learn a lot of things we never knew before about bee venom, honey, cappings, pollen, royal jelly, and propolis.

We're gonna learn about these things in relation to arthritis, neuritis, bursitis, asthma, allergies, ulcers, cancer, cuts, burns, heart disease, frigidity, and rigidity.

We're gonna sleep in the freeway rest areas, the Ozark boonies, next to highballing freight trains, the Detroit Tigers' spring training field, high in the Rockies, two feet from the Atlantic at Key Largo, on Rampart Street in New Orleans, and always, always under the stars.

We're gonna eat catfish, hush puppies, scungilli, turtle steak, Key Lime pie, Montana flapjacks, and lots of Big Macs.

I'm gonna be laying a lot of important stuff on you, but just so I don't overtax your eyeballs I'll be sprinkling some fluff on you now and again for diversion. You can skip the fluff, but not the heavy stuff, because some place in this book is something that will improve your well-being. I promise you that.

OK. Climb up into the van. Now let's git on down the road.

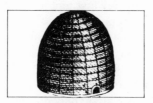

TWO

CHARLIE MRAZ looked about fifty-eight. He was seventy-one. He is a bright, energetic, dedicated man—and obviously successful.

I watched his teenage kids bustle about in the kitchen. I waited my turn while Charlie ministered to a little old lady with arthritis in the knees.

Charlie told me that forty-three years ago he had rheumatoid arthritis and every single joint in his body ached. He had to leave his work in New York City and return to the farm in Middlebury.

All he was able to do was mess with the bees. After several months of this, and many stings, he noticed that all his pains had disappeared except in his knees.

He had a very sensitive spot (trigger point) on each knee, and even the slightest touch would cause sharp pain. It would take him thirty to forty minutes to get from his bed to the kitchen.

Because of the improvement in his other joints, one day he caused the bees to sting both trigger points.

"The next morning I put my feet down on the floor and

walked right into the kitchen. I was so shocked by what I had just done that I couldn't decide whether I had been dreaming I had all this previous difficulty or whether I was dreaming I was cured. That was forty-three years ago, and I've never been bothered since."

Charlie quickly pointed out that this reaction is rare. Usually it takes a great many stings, and the beneficial effect may last only five years. It may last ten or twenty years. However, the treatment can be repeated.

Charlie pressed various spots on both my knees, watching my face for a reaction and looking for sensitive, or trigger, points. He found none.

"Are you sure you have arthritis?"

I told him my GP and an orthopedic man had both assured me that was the problem.

"Do you have it any place else, like your hands or your back?"

I told him my back was OK, but my right index finger sometimes felt like it had been broken and not mended properly and my right hand was stiff for two or three hours in the morning.

He grabbed the middle joint and squeezed it. It hurt plenty.

"Well, that joint's got arthritis in it."

He found a trigger point in my right elbow that reacted like a root canal job when he poked it.

"Doesn't your back get tired after you've been driving for an hour or two?"

With all the style I could muster I told him that I have ridden a motorcycle 800 miles a day without more than four or five "get offs." I was sorry I hadn't claimed something less because I sensed he felt I was putting him on with a claim like that at my age.

"I believe the trouble in your knees stems from your back, and you're going to have to sting your back as well as your knees. I think that in five years you will be seriously afflicted with arthritis. Do you want to try the bee stings or wait or do something else?"

I hesitated a moment. I don't know why, for I had come 3,200 miles for this. I guess the revelation that it probably would take a multitude of stings dimmed my enthusiasm.

"Let's do it," I finally said.

Charlie chilled a small area of my knee with ice, took a bee out of a jar with medical tweezers, crushed the bee's head, and put its tail against my naked knee.

The stinger from the dead bee entered my skin. Charlie removed the bee, leaving the detached stinger with its muscles and poison sac working into my knee. Then quickly he removed the stinger apparatus.

Charlie waited fifteen minutes watching me closely to see if I was having any allergic reaction at any point not contiguous to the stung area. Satisfied that I was not allergic, he numbed two spots on my right knee and applied two more bee stings.

"Sting your right knee one day and your left the next. Start with three stings and increase the stings by one each time until you're stinging yourself between ten and twenty times a day. This jar of bees will last you a few days, and when you come back for more bees bring one of your kids with you and I'll show him how to do your back. And don't drink."

That was Friday, October 1, 1976. On Saturday I got out the jar of bees and some ice cubes to start my own bee stinging or apitherapy (as we "therapists" like to say).

Howsomever, instead of stinging myself I decided to read an eight-page address by Dr. Philip Terc, the father of modern-day apitherapy. I rationalized that would be as good for my arthritis as stinging myself.

Dr. Terc addressed an assembly of beekeepers on February 11, 1904. In part he said:

Years ago I was called to a patient who previously had been treated for rheumatism of the joints, but completely without any success. This lady was not able to move in her bed, suffered in addition with a severe heart disease, and, having heard about bee venom, desperately wanted to try this treatment. After I had examined her very carefully and decided to take the risk, a relative of hers remarked, "Are you actually contemplating to torture this death-bound person?" I first applied one single sting, then after half an hour, two, and after another hour again, two more. She tolerated them well without hardly feeling any pains on application. I stayed for half a day with her to keep her under observation and finally felt entitled to promise her complete recovery. The next day I showed her gardener, a beekeeper himself, how to apply the stings, and three weeks later the "death-bound" patient left her bed for the first time in years. Unfortunately, the patient immediately after having finished the cure, left the district without having achieved full immunization. At the last examination, however, she was not only completely cured of rheumatism but, at the same time, the previous murmur of her heart had entirely ceased.

Dr. Terc used the treatment for forty years. He often said he was convinced that almost all true arthritis and rheumatism can be radically and permanently cured with bee stings, except those cases of many years standing, where the joints already have been destroyed and ossification has taken place.

TABLE SHOWING TERC'S RESULTS

Ailment	No. of patients	No. cured	No. improved	No. unimproved
Rheumatoid heart affections	48	36	7	5
Muscular rheumatism	253	212	41	0
Chronic arthritis	186	151	35	0
Arthritis deformans	17	6	6	5

In 1912 Rudolf Tertch, Terc's son and an ophthalmic surgeon at the University of Vienna, published 660 of his father's cases showing these results:

Perfectly cured	544	82%
Improved	99	15%
Unimproved	17	3%

Sunday, October 3, 1976, I said to myself, "OK, you dummy, you've come 3,200 miles to get some stings—sting yourself." I did, three times, after using ice cubes on the area, and it wasn't bad. It wasn't the funniest thing I've ever done to myself, but it was better than a nail in the foot.

I had decided to sting just my right knee and use the left as a control, since they hurt equally.

I'll be laying some journal notes on you now and again.

Monday, October 4
  Four stings today in right knee.
  Left knee bothers, but not right.

Tuesday, October 5
  Five stings today in right knee.
  Left bothers, but not right.

Wednesday, October 6
  Six stings in right.
  Left still bothers.

On October 7 I ran out of bees, and rather than go all the way to Middlebury I drove to White River Junction to a beekeeper who was also the state bee inspector. We had to wait a bit for him to come home.

Monica and I just lay on the warm grass and watched the maple leaves fall and thicken a carpet the trees were building. Vermont was wearing its fall pajamas.

I've never been able to do much with grass, except cut it. But lying there with the morning sun drawing up the fragrant dew produced an uncommon high in both of us. I even looked forward to getting a new mess of bees.

Mr. William Matson is a quiet, soft-spoken man. I thought he rather suspected my motives, and he was hesitant.

Then he looked at Monica for a long moment. Monica Porter's eyes look like the keyholes to the world's store of compassion and sensitivity. She looks like she may be the mother of nature.

Yes, Mr. Matson said, we could have some bees.

After getting the bees, we visited some and ate apples.

"I knew a young man who had arthritis so bad he had to drop out of college. He went to work for a big beekeeper in Texas that summer. Tended the bees in nothing but shorts and sneakers. Got stung a lot. He came back in the fall with no trace of arthritis, and he never had it since."

Monica and I agreed that was remarkable.

"Even more remarkable to me is the fact that in the twenty-five years I've been an inspector I've never known a beekeeper to die of cancer."

I thought to myself, "Well, I'll be damned!"

These bees were as mean as the owner was gentle. I thought they were gonna come right through the jar to have at me. I tell you I was scared of them.

In trying to get them out one at a time, I fumbled, knocked the jar over, and they poured out in a fury. Fortunately, there was something sweet on the picnic table. Most of them gathered on and around that, and I caught them in a nylon netting that I use for the van windows.

And so on October 7 I stung myself seven times in the right knee. Damn, those bees were mean. My leg started to swell and hurt. I had now had twenty-eight stings. This was the first real evidence of swelling I had had. Healthy people usually swell with the first sting.

Dr. Terc pointed out in his address:

The reluctance of any tendency to swell which I had expected to happen after such a long time, and its finally happening, simultaneously with a very obvious improvement in her rheumatic pains, convinced me more than ever of the peculiar connection that exists between rheumatism and bee venom.

From thereon I gave my special attention to this connection with every new case of rheumatism that came my way. After many years of experience in this line without danger and without sacrifices for an ordinary physician, I found conclusively that people afflicted with true rheumatism do not swell when stung by bees; the number of stings needed to finally bring on a swelling solely depends on the severity and previous duration of the disease. In light cases a few stings will prove to be sufficient. In severe cases, many hundreds or even thousands of stings may be needed until a swelling or secondary reaction can be achieved.

Friday, October 8

Right knee, leg, and ankle swollen way up. Hurts like hell—both painful and numb. Got alarmed and checked the printed material

Mraz gave me, which indicated when you get this reaction the cure's working and it's downhill from here on out.

Saturday, October 9
Knee still hurts.

Sunday, October 10
Not much pain today, but still a lot of swelling and it itched something *fierce.* Took some Alka Seltzer to calm the itching.

Tuesday, October 12
Stung right knee seven times. Swelled and hurt, but not nearly as much as the first time.

Wednesday, October 13
Started with left knee. Three stings. Even the stinging hurt like hell. More importantly, the left knee/leg swelled and hurt a lot after only three stings. Maybe we'll cure this one quickly.

Jan Manley keeps bees. She told me about a knowledgeable beekeeper in South Woodstock, Vermont, who had some interesting tales to tell about bee venom.

"Mr. Wood, my name's Fred Malone, and I wonder if I can come up and talk with you about bees and bee venom."

"All right, come up tomorrow morning if you've a mind to."

"What time's convenient?"

"Well, don't get here before 6:30. What did you say your name was?"

"Malone—Fred Malone."

"Well, five or six years ago there was a Malone running for governor. You be he?"

"Yes, but can I come anyway?"

"Sure, come along."

Clyde Wood told me that in 1935 he became quite ill. The Rutland General Hospital diagnosed Hodgkin's disease. The Mary Hitchcock Hospital in Hanover, New Hampshire, confirmed the diagnosis and advised him to get his affairs in order because there was no cure for Hodgkin's disease. He had about a year, at best, to live, they said.

Mr. Wood checked into a chiropractic clinic in the Midwest and was treated there for about a month.

At the end of the year, when he should have been bargaining with the undertaker, he was aware of two things. He was now immune to bee stings after keeping bees for two years, and his Hodgkin's disease symptoms had disappeared, never to return.

He is seventy-nine now and in excellent health. He is convinced it was either the chiropractors or the bee venom that cured him.

His GP chose to believe it was the bee venom.

Thursday, October 14

Left knee still swollen *sore and tender.*

Gave three-sting "booster" shot *to my right* knee in the PM.

My right *hand* doesn't seem to be stiff when I awake in the morn.

Dr. Terc believed there was a "general effect" as well as a local effect.

Colonel James Vick, a U.S. Army scientist, discovered that bee venom injected into dogs subcutaneously, as the bee does when she stings, sharply increases cortisone production. Cortisone relieves arthritic inflammation.

In Russia, N.M. Artemov discovered that bee venom acts on the body through the pituitary and adrenal glands, stimulating cortisone output.

I must tell you about my friend Bob Richardson. I stayed with him while in Vermont.

Bob is truly one of the kindest, most agreeable men I know. He lives alone and is lonely—which is a small tragedy. He is warm and gentle and would make any one of a hundred thousand lonely women very happy.

We built houses together, we crossed the country on motorcycles together, and we like the same women.

I'm about to put the ice on the spot to be stung, and Bob says, "Fred, I believe it would work a lot better if you would sting yourself without using that ice first."

I did, and hooooeeee it smarted. "Damn—mind your own

business." He didn't offer any further suggestions along those lines.

I advise those of you who are heading for the hives to use the ice until you can't feel it anymore and then apply the sting with dispatch.

It's getting cold in Vermont. Northeastern rains have blown down all the leaves. Let's press south and grab some warms.

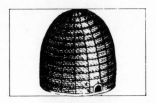

THREE

I SPENT the night in a mowing rimmed by the hills of northern Virginia. It was quiet until morning, and then cows mooed me awake. I was plunk in the middle of a sorority of holsteins. The ladies didn't seem to mind, and after brief pleasantries I rolled south.

Virginia is a beautiful state—manicured, civilized. If the natives seem to be a bit smug, perhaps they have a right to be.

Bob Richardson had suggested I stop by and see a friend of his in Rockwood, Tennessee. He wouldn't give me a letter of introduction or anything as proper and useful as that. He doesn't like to write letters, although he's good at it. He just wanted me to walk right in, bald-faced, with the heavy announcement that I was a friend of his.

Well, I had rid myself of inhibitions early in my prime by riding the Flatbush Avenue trolley at the age of nine. Still, I needed some reasonably comfortable entrée. And so I introduced myself as a special courier with a single red rose from Bob Richardson. You get a lot of mileage from a single rose.

I hope I remain her friend a long, long time.

Joan Smith is a statuesque (whatever that means) redhead with an inordinate amount of zest, instinct, and sensitivity.

When the brains were being handed out, she double-dipped. Joan and her kids run a fishing lodge on Watts Bar Lake, operating from a magnificent slice of lake frontage.

I told her my bee tales. She could hardly contain herself. Since that day in October she has uncovered a whole mess of stuff for me. And she located a nearby beekeeper, for I was out of bees again.

"Here, hold this board," said Mr. Rector, the beekeeper.

The top of the board was covered with bees, and Mr. Rector went to get a bee brush to brush them into my jar.

I clutched that board with hundreds of the little buggers crawling around and mused, "You keep cool, Freddie Boy, cause if you're scared they can smell it. One false smell and you're gonna OD on BV."

"Brother" Tidwell, a fellow beekeeper, stood back and watched with the sly glint of someone about to witness a happening.

Mr. Rector got back before my fear juices flowed, and I was much relieved. I got a couple of dozen bees, a chunk of sassafras limb to make some tea, and the good advice to see Mr. L. Little, beeman, in Shelbyville, Tennessee.

Mr. Little gave me a bunch of good tips on intelligently researching bees and bee venom. He also told me that when he was eighteen he had arthritis so badly in his shoulders that he could not comb his hair. After he had kept bees for a year, it went away. Mr. Little also cured the arthritis in his wife's hands with bee stings.

"I knew a young woman who was so crippled with arthritis she was confined to a wheelchair. Two doctors took her in tow, gave her bee stings, and she was up and about in six weeks," he said.

Mr. Little had been in the bee business full time for fifty years, and he had never known a beekeeper to die of cancer.

He told me about a Dr. Guyton, who treated arthritis with bee venom. He thought the doctor was at the University of Alabama in Tuscaloosa, "If he's still alive." I scurried down to the university at Tuscaloosa and spent the better part of a day looking for Dr. Guyton. No one had ever heard of him.

Bourbon Street in New Orleans is a forsaken street by day. The smells of decaying food; strippers in jeans popping in and out of dark saloons; lightly clad tourists wondering, "Is this all there is?" It's a dismal scene. But nighttime is something else again.

I wandered into Pat O'Brien's for a beer. Two female piano players pounded their machines like they were pumping to save the *Titanic.* They had the crowd singing, clapping, boozing—happy as hell.

Down the street the sweetest jazz I've ever heard was slipping out of Preservation Hall. The "hall" is about thirty by forty feet, jam-packed at a dollar a head. The music seeped through the loose window mullions. Folks were sitting on the floor smiling, and laughing now and again at a mischievous riff. At the corner, under a street lamp, a circle had formed around a black youth who was tap dancing to the jazz pouring from a saloon. He glided around the inside perimeter of the circle with inverted derby in hand and collected a sizable boodle of quid. Bluegrass rhythms thundered down an alleyway like 3,000 buffalo heading for the last salt lick in Montana. I tell you, nighttime Bourbon Street can hone your vibes so your nerves want to spring right out of your bones and play ring-around-the-rosy on the cobblestones.

Rampart Street seemed quiet enough for a good snooze. I checked the door locks several times. I slept quite comfortably. Nobody even pounded on the side of the van.

The next morning, while breakfasting on a Mufletta, I learned that the fifth neighborhood murder in less than a fortnight had befallen Esplanade Avenue, just a couple of blocks away. But the fiend hadn't gotten me, and that was good, for I still had much to do. I built a fire in the box and steamed out of New Orleans through bayou country and land of the sugarcane.

You see a lot of inane, nonsensical official signs while driving across the country. Stuff like "Drive Legally," "Read Signs." Washington has a sign: "Cover on Roadsides Left for Wildlife." I do hope critters have the good grace to take the time to read those signs and are sufficiently appreciative.

Texas has a sign that I snickered at when I first spotted it: "Drive Friendly." And do you know, by God, they do. On a two-lane highway it's common to see a Texan pull onto the shoulder to let an anxious traveler pass. They do that and make lots of other friendly moves. Texans are nice folks.

One day I was driving down a hot ribbon of Texas road when this big mass appeared. "Holy Jeez, what the hell's going on. Duck! Get down! That sumbitch is gonna git us—hell, what is it? Jeez almighty, it's a vulture. It's a goddam vulture!"

I thought I was on a Disneyland set because that must be the only place you find buzzards. It hit my windshield cornerpost and bent my aerial. But it could have been worse. Imagine that —a damn buzzard—oooee, they're ugly rascals.

Across Texas, New Mexico, and Arizona I didn't have any luck getting bees. They're there, sure, but I didn't know where to look for them.

"That's the damnedest thing I've ever heard," Bill said.

I had been spinning my bee tales while we sat around Bill Darrid's pool. I sold Bill some land in Vermont and built him a chalet in 1963. We've been good friends ever since. He uses my hands, and I use his brains. Bill is a writer, a very good writer, very curious, very perceptive. Mrs. Bill is a fine actress, who knows her craft well and enjoys it. She is a foxy lady, good-humored and bright. Her stage name is Diana Douglas.

"Catch some bees and let's see you do it."

I caught some bees, took an ice cube out of the glass, numbed an area, and applied a bee. When I felt the sting I removed the bee. (The bee dies after using her stinger.) The Darrids were fascinated by the stinger working into the skin, independent of the bee. The two barbed shafts of the stinger slide alongside each other, the muscles attached to the top of the shafts thrusting one shaft forward and then the other, and so on. The muscles keep working on their own. They will bury the shaft in the skin if left on the flesh five to ten minutes. The venom is injected between the two shafts. In manipulating one of the bees I caused its stinger to be discharged on my pants. I put the stinger on my knee, barbed points down, and it worked itself right in.

Diana watched transfixed. I explained that I'd rather do it myself, with the live bee, than get an injection at a clinic, even if one were available. Seemed more manly—more natural—like a good and proper collaboration between me and the bee. I even feel there is a sense of sacrificial camaraderie—me and the bee. But perhaps this is a unilateral feeling.

Bill said, "This whole thing looks like a Chinese operetta."

I laughed, and for all I knew it did—I have never seen a Chinese operetta.

It was time to turn north and head for Victoria, British Columbia, and "home." Everything I own, except my motorcycle, is in my van. I have no mailing address, so I use "home" loosely. Everybody has to have a home, according to the rules. Since three-fifths of the people I love are in Victoria, that's home.

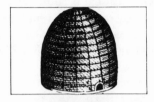

FOUR

"ACCORDING TO the Victoria *Times*, you sell honey. Do you keep bees also?"

"Yes, we have some bees," said the beekeeper's wife.

"I have a touch of arthritis. Do you suppose I can buy a few bees from you for some stinging?"

There was a little chuckle and then, "Sure, come ahead."

Judging by the size of the ad, I figured it would be a two- or three-hive operation tucked underneath an apple tree.

Not so. These folks had 3,000 hives, and this was by far the largest operation I had gotten next to. Each hive has, on an average, 60,000 to 80,000 bees. And 3,000 times 60,000 is a mess of bees!

They collected a "ball" of bees that, by later count, turned out to be well over 400. I was happier than two pigs in the sun.

"Do you or your husband have arthritis?"

"No."

"Did you ever know a beekeeper to die of cancer?"

"No, I don't, but that's how I got into the bee business. When I was twenty-one, I had cancer. I had been operated on seven times. After the seventh operation the doctor told me he was afraid they had done all they could, but they still hadn't gotten it all. As I was going down the path to the car, the doctor's young wife called me aside. She had been working in her flower garden. She said, 'I couldn't help but overhear my husband. You have nothing to lose. Try this. Eat one pound of grapes every day, chew and swallow as many of the seeds as you can, and eat one tablespoon of honey every day.' I did, and I'm sixty-eight now. I still eat a pound of grapes every week and a lot of honey every day. After I had gotten well, I really became interested in bees, got a few hives, and this is what developed. Do you know what propolis is?" she asked.

"No."

"Propolis is a glue made from resins the bees gather from trees and plants. It's a nuisance to a beekeeper, but we sell a batch of it every so often to a pharmaceutical firm in Germany. They do something to it and then use it for people who are allergic to penicillin. Several months ago my husband got an infection where he had just had a tooth extracted. The dentist gave him a prescription for penicillin. Instead of buying the penicillin, that night my husband pushed a bit of propolis onto that infection and in the morning the infection was gone."

Ed Nelson, another Victoria beekeeper, told me some time later that he has used propolis to cure warts and a stubborn fungal infection between the toes.

Here is the *ABC & XYZ of Bee Culture* definition:

Propolis—(from the Greek: pro, before, and polis, city, referring to its use in partially closing the entrance or gateway to the bee commune or city)—Propolis is a gum gathered by bees from a variety of plants, but especially from the buds having some sort of gum or sticky substance. As it occurs in the bee hive, it is from a yellow to a dark reddish brown in color, and resembles a pitch of commerce. It has an aromatic odor similar to that of the buds of the balm of Gilead.

Between October 1 and November 15 I had stung my left knee nineteen times and my right knee eighty-two times. Now, with this new mess of bees, it was time to get down to business.

From November 15 to November 30, I stung myself 171 times on the left knee and 190 times on the right. Toward the end of the month I was stinging myself on one knee thirty times in the morning and on the other knee thirty times before bed.

Within thirty minutes after stinging, there was no evidence I had stung myself except a tiny blood dot where the stinger had gone in. No swelling, no inflammation, no redness. It was obvious that I was now immune to bee venom.

According to Mraz, I should be rid of the arthritis, but I was not, for my knees still bothered me.

Just five bees remained, and it didn't make sense to use so few on my knees. So I stung my right index finger three times on December 1 and two times on December 3. I have not been bothered with pain in that finger since, nor have I had stiffness in that hand since October 14.

Before getting another mess of bees, I went back to my GP.

"Doctor, are you sure I've got arthritis?"

"Yes, I think you have arthritis, and the orthopedic man thinks so too."

"That's wonderful!"

"What do you mean 'wonderful'?"

"Because if I really have arthritis, I know how to cure it."

"How?"

"Bee stings."

My doctor leaned forward in his chair and whispered almost in disbelief, "You going to let yourself be stung by a bee?"

"Yes." I was reluctant to tell him that I had been stung 472 times by bees, fearful he would hustle me to the funny farm.

"Well, I can see you mean business. I'm going to send you to the best rheumatologist in Victoria. He's a good man; you'll like him."

He is a good man, and I do like him. After examining me for an hour and a half, he said, "You don't have arthritis in your knees." The original diagnosis was wrong.

I felt like saying, "Well, I'll be damned—why didn't you bozos tell me that 472 stings ago?"

Instead, I said, "Well, I've been having a lot of trouble with

my back lately. No searing pain, mind you, just a strong ache.
If I'm working, I get it around two in the afternoon, and it's
almost impossible for me to keep carpentering when I do.
Actually it bothers me more now than my knees do. You suppose the trouble can be in my back?"

I was naked as a jaybird.

"Bend over there and touch your toes."

There was a little humor here because I haven't been able
to touch my toes since my last year of lacrosse. But I tried.

"Looks to me like that last vertebra has a worn-out disc.
We'll take some pictures of your back and your hips. And some
more blood tests."

While I waited for the results of the X rays and special blood
tests, I was happy to get a book from the University of Calgary
entitled *Bee Venom Therapy: Bee Venom, Its Nature, and Its
Effect on Arthritic and Rheumatoid Conditions,* published in
New York in 1935.

BODOG F. BECK, M.D.—Author. Jeez, doesn't that have a lilt
to it. Hot damn. Bodog Beck. I believe if I hadn't been fixed I'd
sire another son just so I could name him Bodog. Of course,
Bodog Malone would not conjure up the same exciting imag-
ery of a Bodog Beck. What a name!

The following, taken from the *New York Times,* January 1,
1942, tells its own story:

Dr. Bodog F. Beck of 116 East Fifty-eighth Street, New York, a physician and author, died here today in a convalescent home at the age of
71.

Dr. Beck, who had served for many years on the staff of St. Mark's
Hospital, New York, was long a exponent of "bee venom therapy" for
the treatment of arthritis and rheumatism. He advocated more abun-
dant use of honey in the diet, and operated bee hives at his private
clinics.

He was the author of "Honey and Health," published in 1938, in
which he discussed in detail the medicinal benefits to be derived from
honey. He also wrote "Bee Venom Therapy."

Dr. Beck was born in Budapest, where he was graduated from the
Royal Hungarian University. He served in the surgical department of
St. Stephen's Hospital, Budapest, and later visited well-known surgi-
cal clinics in all parts of Europe.

What a rich find for me. I must confess that my enthusiasm for bee sting therapy was flagging. At this point I knew personally only three people who claimed cures, and two of them were old-time beemen. It was reasonable to assume that they were somewhat prejudiced.

Sure I had "cured" the soreness in my knuckle and the stiffness in my hand, but couldn't that be just coincidence?

No. Here it was in print. A medical man, in New York City, had spent a good part of his professional life curing patients with bee stings. The book was written to persuade the American medical profession to get involved in apitherapy. It is an excellent handbook with step-by-step instructions.

It is tempting to repeat Beck's book verbatim. What follows is some material I have extracted. Remember it's out of context:

Contra-indications have to be carefully considered. It is important, not only to treat cases correctly, but also to select them cautiously.

Kidney involvements, albuminuria and hydrops demand vigilance and discretion. Cases with cardiovascular complications, as a rule, are not very desirable, and if such pathological conditions are advanced, the treatments are absolutely contra-indicated. Of course, watch out for the trio, the "bête noire" of bee venom therapy: tuberculosis, lues, and gonorrhea. Diabetes is generally a contra-indication, but diabetics only rarely require intense treatments, as arthritis among them is exceptional.

All arthritism caused by endocrine imbalance, like climacteric arthritis, arthropathia ovaripriva, etc., does not respond readily to bee-venom treatment, as the progress of the producing causes remains unbroken. Rheumatoid etiology of course is a peremptory requirement.

INDICATIONS

The ailments listed below are amenable to apitherapy:
  Muscular Rheumatism, Myalgia, Myositis, etc.,
  Neuritis, Neuralgia, Migraine, etc.,
  Acute Rheumatic Fever and Endocarditis,
  Acute and Chronic Arthritis,
  Arthritis Deformans,
  Chronic Surgical Inflammation of the Soft and Bony Tissues,

Iritis and Iridocyclitis Rheumatica,
Dermatoses. . . .
I do not wish to omit the fact that bee venom is also used for various skin diseases. As mentioned before, Lautal, a lay beekeeper, successfully used it in eczema, lupus, epithelioma, and leprosy.

In his international search for cancer among beekeepers, Beck discovered one case. That was a man who died of skin cancer in Hawaii.

D. C. Jarvis, M.D., writes in *Arthritis and Folk Medicine:*

I spent two years checking the observation that beekeepers do not have cancer. Charles Mraz, in Middlebury, Vermont, the largest beekeeper in New England, helped me in this study. Together we were unable to find a single case of cancer in beekeepers, or learn of one who had died of the disease. We did find a case of Hodgkin's disease contracted before the man started keeping bees and eating honey. It was cured after he began his new occupation.

Dr. Beck was a kind, patient man and ill-disposed to invective. Yet his book quietly reflects his impatience with his colleagues for not being more receptive to the possibilities of bee venom.

On a personal level, I too suspect that physicians are sometimes fallible.

My mother was very beautiful when I came crying into the world. The hospital bruised her breasts badly trying to get her milk to flow. Her GP strongly advised her to have one breast removed. My father sought a second opinion, which was negative, and fortunately the scurrilous suggestion was abandoned. When my father paid the GP's bill, he only paid half of it. I presume if the GP had recommended a dual mastectomy, my father wouldn't have paid any of it. My mother died at seventy-seven or seventy-nine, and with all her original equipment.

You will recall that Charlie Mraz said no alcohol during the bee treatment. I thought he meant no *serious boozing.* I found that after taking the stings a modicum of Scotch was most agreeable.

Beck had this to say:

Alcohol during the treatments, even in small quantities, is strictly forbidden because it destroys the effects of the venom. This is the reason that alcoholics are just as resistant to the stings as the bees are anxious to sting them. In severe bee-venom intoxication, on the other hand, alcoholization is the best remedy.

Bees don't like people who are juiced up, and such are well advised to stay out of bee yards. I met many, many beekeepers since starting this research, and it's my impression they are either abstainers or drink only very moderately. I have been told that at a beekeepers' convention, setting up a "hospitality room" or bar is foolishness. Beekeepers believe in bees, not booze.

So much for my evening libation.

In the January 1938 issue of *Annals of Internal Medicine,* Drs. J. Kroner, R. Lintz, M. Tyndall, L. Anderson, and E. Nichols, working under the auspices of the Cornell University Medical College, published a report titled, "The Treatment of Rheumatoid Arthritis with an Injectable Form of Bee Venom."

At that time (and perhaps even now) bee venom serum was definitely inferior in potency to the live sting. Nevertheless, here is their conclusion:

1. One hundred patients with rheumatoid arthritis were treated with an injectable form of bee venom (Apicosan) and seventy-three showed improvement. Thirty-five of the patients were markedly improved and thirty-eight moderately improved. There was definite and lasting relief from pain and swelling and a drop toward normal in the corrected sedimentation rate, if previously elevated.

2. The number of injections varied from 6 to 52 over a period of from one to fourteen months. The patients who received on the

average a longer course of treatment showed the greater improvement.

3. In estimating the results obtained from this study of an injectable form of bee venom (Apicosan) for rheumatoid arthritis one is impressed with the definite improvement in the clinical symptoms and the significant drop in the corrected sedimentation index in a large percentage of the patients. It would seem, therefore, that bee venom is worthy of further study.

The concluding statement is quite plain and unequivocal. What happened as a result of this study by this very prestigious conclave?

Nothing.

The *New York Daily News* on March 21, 1938, published an account of the results Dr. Irving S. Cutter had achieved with bee stings. Of 100 arthritic patients so treated, he reported 17 as entirely cured, 18 as practically well, and 38 as moderately helped. That was 73 percent who were improved.

In 1939, Dr. G. W. Ainlay published in the *Nebraska Medical Journal* the results of treating thirty-seven people with bee venom serum.

Of these cases 11 were acute and 26 chronic. The patients were 26–67 years old (61 per cent were over 45 years old). Of these, 16 were completely cured; 16 had relief of pain, lessened swelling, nearly normal function; four were improved and had considerable relief from pain, but there was little change in the swelling and deformities; one case was unaffected. This patient had parathyroid disturbance with muscle and bony deformities.

The *American Bee Journal,* in its January 1977 issue, reprinted an article by Don Ryan that it first ran in November 1954.

Bee sting therapy for arthritis is as old as history. Hippocrates, "father of medicine," tells about it nearly four hundred years before the birth of Christ. European physicians have treated this crippling disease with bee venom down through the centuries. Yet the medical profession in this country waves aside thousands of authenticated cures as old wives' tales.

There is one outstanding exception. Dr. Raymond L. Carey, osteopathic physician and surgeon of Hollywood, California, has been stinging arthritics with bees for 20 years. Evidence of the efficacy of his treatment has been piling up over this long period.

[This reporter] talked to a man in his thirties, an inspector in a precision tool factory [a patient of Dr. Carey's]. John had lost his job. His arthritis had got to the point where he was unable to move his head from side to side. It was rigid on his spine. After two weeks of bee sting therapy John called on his boss. The latter stared open-mouthed while John gave him a demonstration, moving head and neck with swanlike grace. John got his job back.

There is plenty of evidence in Dr. Carey's bungalow that bee venom is a specific for arthritis. But Dr. Carey holds a theory of much greater import. He has not proved this theory. He wishes that some research institute with funds to carry on an extended program, using controls, would undertake the task. This is what he says about it:

"It is my belief that bee venom, through its effects on the central nervous system, stimulates the glands of internal secretion—the pituitary, the adrenal, also the sex glands—enabling the body to utilize its own hormones."

Dr. Carey has recorded numerous cases of painful menstruation normalized by bee venom.

During the course of my visits to the Victoria library, I discovered fifteen arthritis books listed. The card descriptions indicated that eight of these had the theme "learn to live with it," and they were all on the shelves. The remaining seven seemed to have the theme "arthritis can be conquered," and though I looked for eight months, none of the "up" seven were ever on the shelves.

OK, let's now find some people who have cured themselves. Let's find physicians or beekeepers or clinics where people can get help. Let's get some first-hand information that arthritics can understand and lay some options on them.

The results from the back and hip X rays and special blood tests came in, and all were negative. I think I really had those boys stumped because now they wanted to do a biopsy.

Let's git before they start talking autopsy.

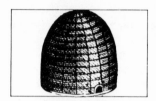

FIVE

"IT'S FAIRLY common that children born of parents who are rather old have a bone missing either from each wrist or from each ankle." Mr. Lange of Mount Vernon, Washington, was speaking to me while he was packaging liquid honey.

I indicated surprise at this news.

"I found that my wrists were getting more inflexible," he went on. "I finally lost all lateral movement in my right wrist. The same thing was happening to my left. The doctor said nothing could be done. It was a form of arthritis and it would get progressively worse. An arthritic customer of mine gave me a home remedy to try. As long as I take it every day, my left wrist remains flexible and useful. When I skip it three or four days, it takes another three to four weeks before I have the good effect again. So I take it every day at breakfast. I've told a number of arthritic customers about it, and about half, I would say, get considerable benefit. The rest don't."

Here's Mr. Lange's recipe:

Mix together the juice of six lemons, two cups of raw honey, one-half cup of Epsom salts. Take a tablespoon of this in hot water every morning. Remember, you must take it every day and it will take about a month to notice good effects, if there are going to be any.

Mr. Lange told me that as a youngster he had run into a partially buried pipe and put a hole in his leg so the bone was exposed.

"It just wouldn't heal. It was a running ulcer. I went to three doctors and then to a specialist. It got to the point where they were talking about amputating. Then a young doctor told me about a preparation his father, also a doctor, used to use. It was honey, castor oil, and a third ingredient. I didn't write it down and I can't remember the third component, but in a little while the flesh came back. I have a little spot there, but it's never troubled me since."

From the *Journal of Obstetrics and Gynaecology of the British Commonwealth,* "Radical Operation for Carcinoma of the Vulva: A New Approach to Wound Healing," by Denis Cavanagh, Chairman of the Department of Gynecology and Obstetrics, Saint Louis University School of Medicine, Saint Louis, Missouri; John Beazley, Senior Lecturer, Institute of Obstetrics and Gynaecology, Chelsea Hospital for Women, London; and Frank Ostapowicz, Chief of Obstetrics and Gynecology, Saint Louis University School of Medicine, Saint Louis, Missouri:

Breakdown of the wound is the most common complication of radical vulvectomy with bilateral groin and pelvic lymphadenectomy. Postoperatively the blood supply to the skin of the groin area is impaired and the healing process is slow. Healing rarely occurs by primary intention and skin grafting may be necessary to assist wound closure. . . .

Recently we have been able to improve wound healing in these patients by local applications of honey. This unusual treatment was first brought to our attention by Professor Scott-Russell of Sheffield during 1968. The method was applied to several infected abdominal wounds in Sheffield and St. Louis.

In our experience honey is much more efficacious than the expensive topical antibiotics which we used previously. The patient's acceptance of the method is excellent once she overcomes her initial surprise at the apparently ridiculous method of treatment. Following discharge from the hospital, patients may easily have the honey applied by a relative or nurse.

With this technique the modal time patients have remained in hospital has been reduced from seven to eight weeks to three to four weeks.

In *Honey and Health,* Dr. Beck writes:

Our good friend, the famous globe-trotter Dr. W. E. Aughinbaugh, described an operation he witnessed in Panama, during the construction of the canal. A native Indian surgeon of considerable repute performed a disarticulation of the hip joint. He smoked cigarettes incessantly during the operation, laid them down occasionally, picking them up again with his bloody fingers. After the stump was sutured, the surgeon took from a large pail several handfuls of honey, which he smeared over the wound, covering it subsequently with gauze. He assured Dr. Aughinbaugh that he had never had an infection when he applied a layer of honey over the wound. Dr. Aughinbaugh has seen the natives of the Amazon region "suture" extensive injuries by letting beetles unite the margins of wounds with their robust mandibles. After the heads of the insects were severed, the mandibles remained closed and the wounds were covered with honey mixed with liquid wax. The results were excellent.

It is singular that, though honey was used for thousands of years for treatment of wounds and skin troubles, our modern medical literature ignores the subject. Lately, it seems, honey is gradually regaining its age-old repute and lost popularity. Dr. Zaiss, of Heidelberg, considers honey in the treatment of wounds superior to all other ointments. He has treated several thousand cases of severe infections with honey and could not report a single failure.

"If I were you, Fred," said Mr. Lange, "I'd stop and see Roy Thurber in Seattle. He knows a lot about bees. Good luck with your book. Tell people about the bees."

I was a little apprehensive pulling Roy Thurber's doorbell. It is a tweedy neighborhood complete with horse paddocks and an inordinate amount of class. It was dark, and I was arriving unannounced. I was sorry he would not see my van when he opened the door because it has fundamental quality.

This fear was unfounded. Always, when visiting with bee-keepers I had the feeling they would willingly interrupt a hot shower to talk bees.

"My mother and father, both grandparents on both sides, and my sisters all have arthritis. I show no signs," Roy Thurber said.

Mrs. Thurber told me she had been taking cortisone shots for bursitis in her shoulders when she started tending the bees. The cortisone wasn't doing her any good, so she stopped taking the shots. After about eight months of tending the bees and getting stung, she lost all signs of bursitis.

I took a "suite" at a rest area on I-5 in Washington. After a bit of hearty burgundy and cheese, I rolled out my four inches of foam rubber, slipped under my eiderdown quilt, and reflected on the day.

I had gotten some significant data from my interviews and the names of a host of people to look up in both the U.S.A. and Canada. The leads Roy Thurber gave me were to prove invaluable. A mosaic was to unfold that even now surprises me. I went to sleep to the rumblings of a diesel truck parked alongside my van.

Mrs. Clarence Wenner took me on a tour of her vegetable garden while I waited for her husband. He had rehearsed the night before with a barbershop quartet and was a little late starting the day. The snow peas were about ready to pick. The Wenners had thirteen employees who gathered around the table at mealtimes—beekeeping in California is big business. Clarence had kept bees for fifty-six years, and he was obviously good at it.

Mr. Wenner didn't have arthritis, and he knew people could be cured by bee stings. He didn't know what the connection between beekeeping and cancer was, but he had never known a beekeeper to die of cancer.

"Yes, I use propolis on cuts and wounds. It always looks clean and good when you use propolis on trouble spots. It's nature's way of overcoming its own defects."

The ABC & XYZ of Bee Culture has this to say:

> Propolis is the base of an important antiseptic preparation used by surgeons. In a hospital where 58 surgical cases were treated with Propolish-in-vasogen (Pearson & Co., Hamburg), there was not a single failure. The results were much less favorable in cases where this preparation was not used. It is highly recommended as a domestic remedy for wounds and burns.

Mr. Wenner has a grandson who is allergic to bee stings. His parents hope to send him to Connecticut to Dr. Mary Lovelace, who has had great success in immunizing people against bee stings.

The Wenners warmed my day even more than the California sun. Old folks are neat folks. The race is over. They're relaxed, mellow, interested in younger people—their ambitions and their foibles. They've rid themselves of the jerkiness and economic kinkiness that plagues us most of our productive years.

It took me three or four stabs before I located Howard Foster's "queen" yard in Colusa, California, and I sure am glad I hung in there. Howard apologized that he was in the midst of working with his queens and couldn't delegate this particular work. He suggested I talk with his wife. This turned out to be a most agreeable suggestion.

Mrs. Foster was practicing the organ for a church recital the next day. I sounded the bell, and a very elegant and intelligent lady asked me in.

"Yes, well, of course, I used honey on my boys' faces for acne all through those difficult years. Clears it right up, you know. And several years ago I had a good friend visit me who was an executive with a leading cosmetic company. I questioned her about a new facial mask they were heavily advertising and whether she thought it would be good for me. My friend advised me the best thing I could use for facial care was plain honey washed off after twenty or thirty minutes with warm water."

Naum Ioyrish writes in *Curative Properties of Honey and Bee Venom:*

Hippocrates remarked on its ability to preserve the beauty of the complexion. Professor M. Bremener, Professor D. Lass, Dr. M. Polikarpova and other authors recommend honey masks as a means with which to strengthen and soften the skin; the masks are made either of pure honey or of a mixture of honey, egg yolk and sour cream.

The most widespread honey mask is made from 100 grammes of honey (if the honey has crystallized, it should be heated), 25 grammes of alcohol and 25 grammes of water. This is mixed until a uniform mass is obtained. This mass is spread in a thin layer over the face (after it has been cleansed with oil) with cottonwool and allowed to stay on for about 15 minutes. . . .

Honey masks are more effective than creams and ointments, because they not only soften but also nourish the skin. Owing to the high hygroscopic properties of honey, it absorbs secretions of the skin, while its inhibitors act as disinfectants.

"I think Hood Littlefield in Visalia was cured of arthritis by bee stings," Mrs. Foster said. "Perhaps you should see him. Also you should talk with my son, Jim. He lives on the next block. He had, or maybe has, rheumatoid arthritis."

I scooted around the block as quickly as I could.

"Jim, your mother tells me you have arthritis."

Jim is maybe twenty-eight, a big Jack Armstrong type, hardly the typical stereotyped arthritic.

"I was working for Boise Cascade several years ago as a draftsman, and making good money, when rheumatoid arthritis hit my hands so badly I couldn't hold a pencil—couldn't function. So they put me on the road, and then I got it in the feet and shoulders. I was going through a tough divorce, not getting much sleep, drinking more than I should. It got so bad I couldn't sleep at night. The doctor told me to take aspirin until my ears rang. I did, and they did. Then they wanted to give me cortisone and gold salts. Almost in desperation, I quit and came to work for my father running bees. Well, I noticed after taking quite a few stings the arthritis didn't seem to bother much. And then I had a little accident with a hive and took a lot of stings. I haven't been bothered since. But it's also true that I eat regularly now, get a lot of sleep, and drink very little. So I don't know—maybe it's the combination. The only time I'm troubled is in the winter when I'm not around the bees."

Howard Foster's father and grandfather were both professional beekeepers. His grandfather died at ninety-seven and his father is alive now at ninety-one. He knew of only one beekeeper who had died of cancer.

All my readers are doubtless aware that health is a very precious commodity. This was brought subtly to my attention in 1963 when I was developing land in Vermont. I owned about 1,000 acres, all of it heavily mortgaged. The economy was down. We hadn't had any real rain for two years, and the prospect of forest fires was imminent. A careless match and I'd be wiped out.

The late Frank Mylott worked for me then clearing brush at a $1.50 an hour. He knew I might be building an ulcer. "Never worry about anything you can buy or sell," he told me. It probably was the most valuable advice I've ever been given. I never did get an ulcer.

"Never worry about anything you can buy or sell." Anchor to that thought. It may save your life.

"Dr. Laidlaw, sorry to be phoning you at this time of day. Roy Thurber suggested I call. I'm doing research on bee venom and arthritis."

"I cured the arthritis in my wife's hands with bee stings, but if you really want to find out about bee stings and arthritis, get in touch with Professor Guyton in Alabama."

"I thought Dr. Guyton was dead."

"No, no. He's very much alive and living in Auburn, Alabama."

"Hot damn," I said to myself. I talk to myself a lot.

Dr. Laidlaw is an entomology professor emeritus at the University of California. He suggested I check the college library.

The library was a little difficult for me to master. In fact, I secreted myself in an alcove so well that I darn near got locked in for the night. I just did find my way to the front desk by the six o'clock closing. On Sunday I left a trail of cookie crumbs so I wouldn't risk ensnarement again.

I found the book I had been seeking for months: *Bee Venom,* by Joseph Broadman, M.D. published in 1962. Dr. Broadman describes his technique and gives case histories. He mentions dozens of clinics in Europe in which bee venom therapy is used for arthritis and other ailments.

Please remember that in some instances the following extracts have been taken out of context:

Resistance to bee venom as a curative has been strong in America, and it is strange that one of the most advanced countries in the world allows millions to go in agony and be crippled unnecessarily; even worse, almost all of the medical profession is completely ignorant of what been venom can do and has done.

It is this resistance and ignorance that has forced me to write this book.

In my office, a hundred people, after relief from arthritis and rheumatism, have said to me, "Why doesn't everyone know about this treatment?"

My answer is usually one of despair and some anger. For years I have tried to publish articles in medical journals all over the country. Two have been published, but recognition for the honey bee is slow. Recently, the American Cancer Society published an article in *Cancer News* called "Does a Honey Bee Have an Answer to Cancer?" And it was gratifying to note that the Society is now doing research on the honey bee's venom, even for a disease outside of my immediate professional interests.

For most readers who are personally involved with arthritis or rheumatism, I tell you that a solution to your problems is within your grasp. It is your right to be free from pain and crippling transformations. You must demand that freedom—even if you have to "educate" your doctor to get it. . . . Synthetic steroids have proved defective in the treatment of arthritis and rheumatism; in fact, steroid hormones such as cortisone, ACTH, Butazolidin or their derivatives have under scrutiny been challenged as practically useless by many specialists in the treatment of arthritis and rheumatism. Further, these drugs are dangerous, often causing serious side effects or death. They do not cure; neither doctors nor drug manufacturers claim they cure.

It is not the province of this book to belabor the dangers inherent in cortisone and allied drugs. However, a multitude of medical apitherapy practitioners state that the *only* side effects of bee venom observed have been an increased feeling of well-being and an improvement in general health.

Working under the Food and Drug Administration's New Drug Application DBS-IND-292 for testing the toxicity of bee venom, W. A. Benton stated in September 1971: "It was concluded that honey bee venom at the level injected (up to 12 mg/week) had no adverse physiological or mental effects."

Now back to Dr. Broadman:

I managed to achieve publication in only one medical journal in the United States (*General Practice* . . .). Then all avenues closed for future articles on bee venom. The first article was mailed to nearly every medical journal in the country. Two or three responded favorably, but did not publish the article. One journal accepted, only to return the article to me near publication time. The explanation: two members of the editorial committee, who were especially interested in arthritis and rheumatism, "objected" to its publication.

The medical profession received Dr. Broadman's book with somewhat dimmed enthusiasm. One of the Arthritis Foundation's local chapters characterized the book as a "quack item." Dr. Broadman sued for $2.5 million, and they settled out of court. More on Dr. Broadman later.

"I was aware that there was some value in bee stings for helping arthritis," Jack Jensen said, "but I wasn't aware that the treatment needed to be local."

Jack and I were bouncing down the South Plow Camp Road in Los Banos, California. The CB radio in the pickup cut in periodically. "I couldn't understand why in the summer when I was doing all this lifting I'd never be bothered, and in the middle of the winter I'd come down with this thing. I come down with it last January, and for ten months . . . I couldn't do anything—nothing. I couldn't even ride around in a pickup and not be suffering. It's high in my spine. There's a reason for it: I broke my spine as a youngster.

"I went to doctors. I was scheduled for a myelogram and a look-into surgery. This kept up in my mind: Why do I get the pain in the middle of winter? People say it's cold weather. Well, I'm an avid deer hunter, and we go out of state and sleep in the snow and really rough it in October and November in zero weather and the arthritis never bothers me. I come home to a nice environment, and for three years in a row it's been the same time, the week between Christmas and the first of the year.

"The last week of December, working on the books, closing the books. I'd sit at a desk for about two hours and I'd go to get up and I couldn't get up. The pain would lock me up. This year it just got worse and worse—muscle spasms. Really it was the worst time I ever spent in my life. I went to a chiropractor. I went to a medical doctor, who gives arthritis treatments."

I asked if the doctor had given him gold salts.

"No, it's a local doctor here in town. He gets the serum from horses—I don't really know the term or name of it or what. He's treated a lot of people, and he's had fair success. I mean it don't work on maybe 40 or 50 percent of the people. In my case he could see that break, and there was a little arthritis, but it didn't look like enough to cause the kind of trouble I was having.

"In fact, one day I had a spasm in his office, and he couldn't believe it. My back muscles would draw me backward till I just tipped over—unbearable. So anyway, a friend told me about a doctor friend of his who gave acupuncture treatments. He said, 'Why don't you try this?'

"So I went to that doctor. It was the first relief I can say I got. I took acupuncture treatment from him for about four months and I progressively got better. But the pain was still there, and if I did any real physical work, I'd suffer."

The CB cut in, and Jack talked with one of his men for a while.

"Well, this article in the bee journal come out about two months ago, and that was the first time I knew the treatment had to be right on the spot. Over the winter I had been letting the bees sting me on my hand because I thought you just had to let the venom get in your system. So about a month and a half ago I started giving myself stings right on the area, and it's just unbelievable. I mean the arthritis just cleared right up. As far as I'm concerned it's just a miracle."

We got back to the house and Jack invited me in for coffee.

"Two winters ago, I had a real bad attack, but it was short. Lasted maybe a week. I'd be down, generally, maybe three or four days bad, and then it would gradually clear up and I'd be completely over it, but this lasted longer than usual. Then in May, I had another little deal. I was irrigating and I did so much shoveling. The attack didn't last long and it wasn't as severe.

"But the pain was still with me. Then I went out and unloaded a load of bees, and I had an accident. About seven hives fell off one side of the truck. Boy, the bees really worked me over. It's been a long time since I've been stung that bad. I remember my shirt pulled up out of my pants and a dozen bees stung me all up my back. I never had a bit of trouble all the rest of that summer. I look back at this now, to see if there's a correlation, you know. I believe there is—like I say, it's just been a real great thing with me."

Jack paused for breath, then said: "It's funny, Hood Littlefield—I don't know if you know him."

"I'm on my way down to see him now."

"He had great trouble with arthritis, and his doctors advised him to get a couple of hives and get into the bee business."

I liked Jack Jensen, and I really didn't want to finish my coffee and git. But Visalia is a fair shoot from Los Banos, and I didn't want to be late for my appointment with Mr. Littlefield.

In one respect I chose the worst time of the year to do this research, because I arrived the same time as the bloom in every area of the country.

My introductory remarks were usually: "I'm Fred Malone. I'm doing some research on bee venom and arthritis. You suppose we can visit for a couple of minutes?"

The usual reply was: "You've caught me at the worst possible time of the year. Can you come back in a couple of weeks?"

"No, I'm just passing through this one time."

"Well, OK, I guess I have a couple of minutes."

Two or three hours later, I'd say, "I better git on down the road. I've taken enough of your time."

And the reply was usually, "I can talk bees all day. Tell people about the bees and good luck with your book."

I've done some good stuff and some mischief. The three good things I'll tell you about now and again as we go down the road.

December 26, 1971, I was in the Springfield (Vermont) Hospital at 3 A.M., waiting to see my mother. My mother was a dear, sweet lady. But of course you know that. Thumbing through an old *Mechanics Illustrated,* I came across a saucy sixteen-foot sailboat called a Mediterranean caique, known to you non-Egyptians as a dhow. The article said it was easy to build and sailed beautifully. Part of that was true.

I built it in the back of my real estate office, which was a large Victorian gingerbread house. I could hardly wait till the end of the day to climb out of my broker's uniform and into my carpenter's apron. Working with my hands does magical things for me. I suppose it's because I'm creating. It vaporizes the heaviness in my chest.

I once heard that more of our brain is given over to the movement of the hands than to any other part of the body. Maybe that's why people smoke too much—to pacify that part of the brain which demands action. I've often wondered if that blue funk mothers go into when kids hit their teens isn't caused by a sudden lack of demand on their manual creativity. Their kids don't require constant mothering anymore. After fabricating creations of some merit and nurturing those creations for eight or twelve years, mothers don't have much to do and feel unneeded. Now is the time for them to beat hell out of some clay, paint up a storm, join a woodworking class, learn to weave cloth, knead some whole-wheat dough, and get those hands to making stuff—not driving a ball or popping the old vodka down or joining a bridge club to whine collectively about their voids.

When I finished the sailboat, the *Finbar Xavier Oremus,* I had a launching party of about fifty friends. There were hot dogs, hamburgers, beer, and soda pop for the kids. I was standing on the beach of Lake Saint Catherine with the *Oremus* quivering on a trailer, ready for her maiden voyage.

I had visions of the boat sliding to the bottom like a heavy china plate. I had been on television twice, but the nervousness I felt this day far exceeded the TV jeebies. I believe I was trembling. Bill Darrid put his arm around me. "It's going to be all right, Fred. Not to worry."

It didn't sail worth a damn. But it didn't leak either. It probably brought me more pure joy than a store-bought fifty-foot ketch.

Mr. Littlefield was an hour late arriving for our appointment at his bee "ranch." He apologized, saying that the hydraulic lift on his truck broke down, and he had to lift all the hives off by hand. A hive may weigh eighty pounds or more. I wished I could have helped him.

The blossoms were on the almond trees. Bees are the only way almond trees get pollinated, and the bees must be there when the bloom is on. Mr. Littlefield hadn't had time to get the lift fixed—and he was tired.

I set up my "dining room" in the van, brewed a little phony coffee, and cut some apple crumb cake my lady had baked.

"Well, I had my problem in '44 and '45," he began, "and the doctor in Pasadena advised me to go into the bee business. I was off work for a major oil company at the time because of arthritis in my back."

"Was that Dr. Carey?"

"No another doctor."

"Did you ever talk with Dr. Carey?"

"Oh, yes. Lots of times."

"What sort of man was he?"

"He impressed me as being a real good man. He was a modest sort of guy. He told me he had cured better than 90 percent of the people who had come to him. I'd been to four doctors trying to find out about my problem before my regular doctor came back from the service. I'd been fooling with one hive of bees as a hobby.

"When he told me I was going to have to do something else, I said I didn't know what else to do. I'd never done anything but work for an oil company and try and play ball.

"He was standing there looking out the window, waiting for the time to elapse on the electrical diathermy, and he asked me what kind of hobby I had. I said, 'I guess if I have a hobby now, it's a colony of bees.'

"He turned around right quick and said, 'That's it. Bee stings have helped a lot of people with your problem. Can you get into it to make a living?' And I said, 'I don't have any idea if I can or not.'

"I went home and told the missus. She became an astronaut right quick. She went right through the ceiling."

"Well, did you just go out to your hive and let yourself get stung, or did you purposely put stings on you?" I asked.

"Purposely put stings on me—mostly on my shoulders. The first load I moved after the doctor advised my going in the bee business, we had an accident. Fifteen hives fell off the back of the truck, right in the middle of the road. We went and unloaded the rest and came back and picked the fallen hives up a couple of hours later. There was still a mess of bees. Of course, that was preinsecticide days when we really had bees in the hives. When we came back, we tied our britches' legs down and I wore gauntlets. I never was one to wear gloves, but I had on a pair that night. We'd pick up a hive and set it on the truck till we got all fifteen on. We left a pile of bees there.

"When I got home next morning, a little after eight o'clock, I pulled off my clothes and I was just as red as I could very well be from the bees going in."

"They go in no matter what you do, don't they?"

"Yeah. I thought that would be a good day to go to the doctor —he still had me come for electrical diathermy—so I went, and pulled off my shirt. He looked at me and said, 'I didn't tell you to get all this at one time. Wonder you weren't killed. What happened anyway?' I told him.

"Since that time I've never had any trouble with my back whatsoever. But I did have lots of trouble with my shoulders. I just go out to the beehives when this bursitis gets to where I can't operate. I go out and put a dozen on me and let them run their course."

"Do you know any other people who have been helped by bee stings?"

"Thelma had arthritis in a joint in her finger and the doctor that advised me to go into the bee business told her if she'd put a bee sting on there, it'd take the arthritis away. She had nerve enough to do it, and the arthritis went away and it's never come back. She helps me with the bees. Now she's got so much poison in her when she gets stung it kills the bees."

"Again, I apologize for taking your time today."

"I hope it will help somebody. I hope our roads cross again," Mr. Littlefield said as he waved me away.

I notice you're squirming around in your seat a lot. Your bum must be getting tired with all this driving. Tell you what to do—learned this from riding my motorcycle coast to coast. Sprinkle some Johnson's Baby Powder in your shorts when you're getting dressed tomorrow. Cuts down the friction. Fix you right up.

Bill Darrid and I were going to get a few sticks of wood to build a bookcase. I had told him how I'd been troubled the last several years with cold sores and nothing seemed to work. Remembering that I had read nothing can live in honey because of its tremendous absorptive power, pulling the moisture out of any organism, I had put a little honey on a cold sore (fever blister) one day and the sore had disappeared within hours. And honey has cleared up every one I've gotten since.

"You suppose that would work on canker sores?" Bill wondered. "I've got one that's bothering the hell out of me."

I pulled the van over to a parking meter, fetched a tablespoon of honey out of my pantry, and gave it to Bill.

About half an hour later we arrived home, and I asked Bill how the canker sore was.

"I'll be damned! It's gone."

I tried honey on a canker sore several weeks later and the sore disappeared.

A little while after that I was telling the story to Dr. George Vogel one Sunday afternoon at his house. He jumped up and grabbed the phone in the kitchen.

"Yes, this is Dr. Vogel. Does your daughter still have all those canker sores? Give her three teaspoons of raw honey every day and let me know how she makes out."

The daughter had had a mouthful of canker sores for weeks and couldn't get rid of them. Later Dr. Vogel told me that the following Tuesday the mother called to tell him the canker sores had disappeared.

I wrote a postcard to my friend Bob Richardson telling him to use honey on his next cold sore. He told me the day the card arrived he had a cold sore. He put honey on it and it disappeared in a matter of hours.

It not only works for me, it tastes considerably better than Campho-Phenique.

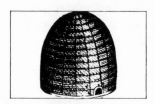

SIX

THE ARTICLE I had read in the *American Bee Journal* mentioned that Dr. Carey had learned his technique from Bodog Beck. Beck had died thirty-five years ago, so it seemed unlikely I'd find Dr. Carey alive now. I checked the phone books and the city directories in the Los Angeles area, fairly certain he would not be practicing, but hopeful I would find him still living in the area. He wasn't.

But I did find him living about four blocks from my kinfolk at Huntington Beach. Just thumbing through a phone book, I found him.

Dr. Carey is eighty-four, white-haired and robust, although he has a touch of emphysema. He lives in modest circumstances a block or two from the Pacific. He and Mrs. Carey (who introduced him to the possibilities of bee venom in Mexico) could not have been more cordial.

Here is just some of what I learned in two days of visits.

"I got a kick yesterday. I was waiting for my wife, sitting in the car. And I turned on the radio. Leonard Pinario, an internationally famous pianist, was announced as the next artist to be heard. I got to dreaming back to the day Leonard came to me with arthritis in the shoulder. The doctor in Rome had X-rayed it and said, 'You have arthritis, you'd better go back to America. Nobody can do anything for it, but you'd better go back anyway.' So he came back here with his prestige, his name, his money, and tried a couple of the people back East. Nothing helped, so he came to me."

"How did he hear about you?"

"Through his mother, who had a friend whom I had treated. So damned if he wasn't able to go back and play the piano in three weeks! Now that's fifteen years ago, and he's still a concert pianist. He came back a year later, and I had the shoulder X-rayed exactly as it had been done a year before, when little spicules of bone could be seen in the shoulder joint. They had completely disappeared. So when they say, 'Does it absorb the calcium?' I have pictures that show the definite absorption of calcium. But that doesn't mean it happens in every case."

Dr. Carey had rummaged in a file cabinet and brought back a thick box of brown-and-white photographs.

"Joe Ground, Conrad Hilton's associate, an old football fan, had hurt his knee, and they were going to operate on it. He came in one morning around nine o'clock. He had arthritis in the knee and the doctors wanted to operate on it. He said he had heard I could help arthritis without operating. I said, 'I think I can.' 'Well,' he said, 'let's go. They want to charge me $2,500 for the operation. What do you charge for bees, $2,500 too?' 'Not yet,' I said.

"Anyway, I treated him three times. Every other morning on his way to the office he'd stop. At the end of the week he didn't have a pain in his knee. And he hasn't since, to my knowledge."

Dr. Carey shuffled around in that photo box for a little bit.

"You know the chap who plays Fred in the 'I Love Lucy' series? His name's Bill."

"Frawley."

"Yes, that's it. Well, Bob Cobb owned the Brown Derby and his mother was a patient of mine, and his sister. He was going with a girl named Sally Wright, a beautiful creature. Sally would come down with Bob's mother when she came in for a treatment, so I got well acquainted with Sally. Bob's mother responded well, but I couldn't do much with his sister.

"However, one day Sally brought Bill Frawley to me because he couldn't raise his arms up. I put three bees on his shoulder and told him to put his shirt back on.

"He said, 'Sally help me with this shirt.' So she helped him. He said, 'Well God damn, Doc—look here. Look how I can move these arms.' He threw a twenty-dollar bill down and said, 'Will this take care of it?' I hadn't had a twenty-dollar fee since I treated an oil millionaire. I was lucky to get three dollars for a treatment. Anyhow, Bill got better."

"And that's all it took, just those three bees?"

"Yes, that was the only time I ever treated him."

"Was it arthritis or bursitis?"

"Neuritis."

I told Dr. Carey how I had initially become interested in bee venom therapy with my gouty friend Ray Murdoch back in Vermont. I asked him if he had ever had any experience with gout.

"Yes, quite a bit. I remember a Frenchwoman. She was a very devout Catholic, on her knees praying most of the time, but she couldn't pray anymore because her knees hurt too much. She knew my father-in-law years ago and she came to see me. I looked at her knee. So help me, under the skin you could see the white chalklike substance—and in the skin, not below but in it. So I told her, 'You know if we put some bees on those knees we may be able to soften that stuff up and get rid of it.' She said, 'Fine.' It didn't seem to hurt her much. Maybe just a little bit.

"It must have been about a week later, after two or three treatments, the redness and heat disappeared. One morning about eight she called me. Said she wanted to come right over to show me something. She came over with a cup of what looked like toothpaste. She said, 'This came out of my knee during the night. Got all over me. Woke me up.'

"The skin had ruptured and these gouty crystals came out of that wound just like toothpaste out of a tube. I called my wife in to look at it. She was shocked."

"There's no other way to get that out?" I asked.

"None known to man. And you can do it every time. Until the day she died she was able to get down on her knees and pray."

We both agreed that the bee is an amazing creature and has secrets we may never discover.

"For instance, I had a case of Buerger's disease. Now, there's no treatment except amputation."

"What is that, Doctor?"

"Beurger's? The inner lining of the arteries hardens. The foot (that's usually what's affected) turns black, gangrenous. We don't know the cause for sure. Poor circulation. But this man was an artist from Russia—a splendid, intellectual man. He'd been in Cedars of Lebanon Hospital and they told him there was no cure for it. He had heard about me some way or other and came to me one day and said, 'Doctor, will you please put bee stings on? I've been told the only answer is amputation and as a matter of fact, on account of my heart, they won't operate.'

"I said, 'Take off your slipper.' He had the top cut off because of the pressure, and he had crutches. He had difficulty getting into my office because at that time I was on the tenth floor of the Transamerica Building with a hive of bees in my window.

"He had a hole in his foot under the first toe. It was dry, gangrenous, and I thought, 'Oh my God!' His feet were like ice. They were half black. He had been under the care of the best orthopedic men, and I'd have a lot of guts to dare to try bee sting therapy, but yet it was a challenge. After a little debate, he said, 'Please do it, Doctor.' I said, 'I don't think I'll be able to help you, but if you insist I'll put a bee or two on you, and if you're no worse tomorrow come on back.'

"Now as true as I'm sitting here talking to you, I put one right next to that sore. He never batted an eye. I looked at him, and watched the bee pump. He said, 'Put another one on.' I put one on the opposite side of the hole.

"You may believe this or not. He put his stocking and his slipper on, he stood up, and he looked at me and said, 'Doctor, please believe me. The pain is less than when I came in and I can feel the blood rushing down into my foot, just pounding down in there.' He could feel every heartbeat. Well, it scared me, so I said, 'You go on home and if you feel good enough tomorrow, come back.' So he left the office and I was glad to get rid of him because, remember, he had suffered from a bad heart, a bad prostate, and this endarteritis—three very difficult things. I was on the tenth floor of the office building, and if anything had happened, I'd be known forever."

"That's right. Never mind the good."

"Never mind the good you do; it's the harm you might do. Well, in five minutes, damned if he wasn't back in the office. I looked up at him and thought, 'Oh my God, what's happened?' He just grinned and said, 'Put some more on me, Doctor, I feel so different, so good!' I said, 'Please get out of here, and stay out for a day until I see what happens. You scare me.' And he did. I was scared to death.

"I had never treated a case like that. I didn't have a right to, but I foolishly went ahead without knowing what I was doing.

"He came back the next day. Three months later he came to my new office and home I had built off La Brea—three dollars a square foot for construction in those days, and I put my beehive in there. Down he comes walking with shoes on, my good friend Boris, and the wound had completely healed. He was feeling like a million dollars. His blood pressure had gone from 247 to 160. The foot had completely healed without a scar, and he was able to walk without pain."

"How many stings had you given him, Doctor?"

"Maybe he had 150 or 160."

"Just two or three each time?"

"No, we got up to six to ten at a time."

"Were you ever worried about malpractice suits?" I asked.

"Yes, constantly, and wondered that I never got one."

Beck, Broadman, and some Russian authors claimed migraine could be helped by bee venom. I asked Dr. Carey about this.

"Did you ever use bee venom to control migraine? I have read in several papers that that works."

"No. I have found that vitamin E, 400 milligrams, is very

efficacious in some cases of migraine headaches. I've known some of my patients it's helped."

"That's good to know. I'll pass it along."

Rona Brown is a delightful retired schoolteacher living in Fordwich, Ontario. She told me some interesting stories of a woman in Ontario who can massage away cataracts using sage honey. Dr. Carey had this to contribute:

"I've had cataracts clear up with honey in the eye."

"You have?"

"Absolutely—and that's another one I don't talk about."

"Do you dilute it with water?"

"No. Put a drop of honey in each eye at night. Let the eye burn, sting, and cry for a little while. Leave the honey in all night long. The tears dilute it, you know. In the morning wash it out with warm water.

"A woman who could no longer sew, thread a needle, or read a newspaper went to her ophthalmologist and was told he wouldn't operate until the cataract was enlarged more. This is twenty-odd years ago. Three weeks later, after the honey treatment, she could read the newspaper and thread a needle. Three months later the doctor could not see any evidence of the cataracts he had diagnosed three months previously, and he couldn't believe it. When the woman told him what she had done, he said, 'Oh, that's nonsense.' "

"Did you use any particular kind of honey?" I asked. "I've read that in Russia and in Ontario, they use sage honey for cataracts."

"No. Just honey. Honey is hygroscopic, draws fluid out. Now, I can't say this from a chemical or a pharmacological standpoint, but it's my opinion that honey does the same thing as pilocarpine, which is used to stop glaucoma by drawing the fluid out from behind the eyes. The patient will cry and weep, and his eyes will sting and hurt at first, but the next morning he can wash the honey out with plain warm water, and improvement starts immediately."

The doctor paused for a moment like he was trying to pull something out of his memory box and then said, "Did I tell you about the baker who had a nasty boil on the back of his neck?

No? Well, he came to me about four o'clock in the afternoon —this is a neighborhood merchant—and he had the nastiest carbuncle; it was developing several heads. I looked at it and, oh boy, was it angry! But it hadn't come to a head. I was told never to do surgery until a carbuncle was ripe; otherwise it might spread.

"I suffered for him the minute I saw him. I could see he was in pain. 'I can't lance this today,' I told him, 'but I'll tell you what we can do so that maybe I can lance it tomorrow.' I said, 'When you get home dip some gauze in honey and put it right over the area. Cover it so the honey won't run over you and get messy. Just make a plaster of honey and gauze and cover the boil and come back tomorrow and see me.'

"The next day he came back, and with a big grin he greeted me. 'I took a half a jar of honey,' he said, 'and soaked the gauze and got honey all over me. I went to sleep because I was relieved and I felt that damn thing rupture and I didn't know whether the honey was streaming down my neck or the pus from the carbuncle.'

"I took the stuff off that he had put on, and that sore was as wide open as the mouth of a child looking for milk. And it was clean as a boar's tooth. Every iota of that nasty sore had been pulled right out—pus, the core—just the crater was left.

"So I said, 'Do it again.' The boil cleared all up, and in a week it was gone."

Another faded photo came out of the box.

"The Reverend Charles Sheldon wrote a book, *In His Footsteps*—world-famous, more copies were printed than of any book except the Bible, up to that time. He was a Congregational minister in Topeka, Kansas, and his wife had arthritis in the shoulders, neck, and arms terribly bad. So he went to the Mayos and they told him there was nothing they could do. Then he wrote to Beck in New York, and Beck told him to come to California and see me.

"Sheldon was a big, white-maned, handsome old gentleman about eighty. He had been a member of Ford's Peace Ship, very well-known throughout the country. His wife couldn't comb her hair, couldn't put her hat on—very charming woman. So I started to treat her. They could only remain two weeks, and I told him I didn't know whether I could do much in two weeks, but I'd try. I treated her every day—Saturday, Sunday, and Washington's birthday.

"After the third treatment she was able to sleep through the night. He was terribly happy about it. She had a pretty good local reaction, incidently—it frightened her, but she kept coming. At the end of two weeks, she could comb her hair. But they had to go back to Topeka. On the way back they stopped to see a doctor friend, and when he heard about me and my bees, he told them they were out of their minds. He said I could have killed her. The Reverend said, 'Well we may be out of our minds and he might have killed her, but he didn't, and she's free from pain and able to raise her arms. This is marvelous and we're happy.'

"A year later he wrote to Beck to thank him for referring them to me because his wife had recovered so beautifully. He said he had asked a number of doctors in Topeka why they didn't use bee stings in arthritis and got no good reasons why not, just excuses. He concluded by saying that if he were a young man he would get a medical degree on purpose so he could use bee stings to treat arthritis. That was the famous Reverend Charles Sheldon. Lovely man."

The doctor coughed a little, left the kitchen table for a few minutes, and was back with a modicum of brandy for us both.

"Rosie Rosenbloom was bent over tragically with spondylitis, and I treated her for considerable time. Charity case—county home. One day she came in and said, 'Dr. Carey, I can see airplanes.' She hadn't been able to look up in the sky to see airplanes in years.

"This created havoc at the county home, where I was an intern, because the doctors knew me and they'd laugh like hell at me. I sent Rosie back to them. They'd been treating her for two or three years, with no results; she was getting worse, of course. When she got better and could see airplanes, I was delighted. I told her to go back and show the boys how she could see airplanes now. As a result they'd send me their worst patients, their incurables—and I got the worst there was.

"I remember one patient with spondylitis—stiff as a ramrod, bent over. He was working for Douglas, I think. He was about to lose his job. He asked for my help, and we started treating him. He started to get better and within six months he was promoted to foreman. His name was Symanski—Polish—hell of a nice kid. Now that's satisfaction. I'm proud to be able to look back and know I helped those people.

"And I can get mad, by the same token, to think you'll be laughed at when you say these things when you know damn well you've done them."

I felt a warm glow. Maybe it was the brandy.

"Then there's osteomyelitis. Very interesting case. Cleared up beautifully. This child was only a boy of fourteen, as I recall. He'd been horribly crippled by all the surgery as well as the affliction, and his osteomyelitis cleared up beautifully after 150 stings."

"Is that right? Did you just treat him locally?"

"Just right on the heels and on the hips. When he came to me there were two holes, muscles coming out of both of them. He had been to several of the Shrine Hospitals; his hips had been frozen and operated on; a joint had been removed. He had fallen out of a tree originally and injured himself. No parents—just an orphan. So I didn't get paid. It didn't matter."

Back about twelve years ago I got bursitis in my hip so badly that I was confined to bed for three weeks. I determined during that time that they could have my leg if that's what it took to get rid of the pain. And that I would sell my motorcycle because I thought I had gotten this from riding with my legs spread-eagled a long time on a very hot day. When I get the slightest pain in a hip now, I become almost unglued with apprehension.

"Did you ever cure bursitis?" I asked Dr. Carey.

"Bursitis, yes. Usually with one or two treatments."

"Did you ever fail to cure bursitis?"

"Really, no. No, I think bursitis is simple. I've always figured it was."

"I'm sure glad to hear that."

"Oh, yes, before I forget it. I had a patient with a lime burn from plaster that had eaten down to the bone of his ribs on his chest, saturated with pus. He came to me—I don't know why or how. I took one look at it and thought, 'My God, this is terrible.' So I said, 'Get up on the table. I'm going to try something new on you.' So I took some honey I had in the office and cut strips of gauze, saturated them with honey, and laid them across this wound. I put a covering over that. Do you know that in three weeks that damn thing was healed and never left a scar? Nothing but honey."

I asked Dr. Carey if he had ever compiled what he thought was his rate of success using bee stings.

"No, and I'll tell you why I never wrote or compiled anything to speak of. Mostly because I never kept the diagnoses in such a way that I could prove what I was doing. When people came to me for help, they were in pain and deformed."

"You weren't experimenting."

"No. I'd treat them to help them. They couldn't afford X rays, blood tests. They were poor—90 percent of them. All I could do was say, 'Look, I think I can help you. If you want me to treat you, I will. If you can pay me, pay me; if you can't, OK.' I didn't want to be a charitable institution necessarily, but I had to be sometimes.

"I was in it for about forty years. I treated a hell of a lot of arthritics. I estimate that I used pretty close to a million bees. Maybe that's an exaggeration, but I don't know. I would see twenty or thirty patients a day, putting on anywhere from 2 to 150 bees apiece. It doesn't take long to get into the hundreds and thousands before you know it.

"And in all that time I never had a bad reaction. One time a doctor had a pretty severe local reaction—a medical doctor who suffered with arthritis came to me for the same reason others did. He had tried everything else. He wanted too many stings. He thought if one is good, two is better; if five is good, ten is better. So one day he came in and said: 'I want twenty-five of these things. I'm feeling fine.' I said, 'No, twenty-five is too many.' 'Oh, hell,' he said, 'there's nothing to these things.' And foolishly I let him get away with it. He had a pretty severe reaction. Not true anaphylaxis, but he broke out in a sweat and fever, redness and itching, shortness of breath. But he recovered quickly. And his arthritis went away. He didn't require any more treatments.

"Now there's an interesting thing I've never been able to prove: When they get a severe reaction, they get well that much faster. And yet you're scared to death to build up to that reaction. Now if you were in a hospital where you had the facilities for emergencies—respiratory aids, oxygen, adrenaline—which you might use, you could afford to take more chances. This way, people come off the street, go out, get in their cars, and drive off, and you're taking a hell of a chance.

"I've never been able to carry insurance. It's not accepted treatment."

"They wouldn't insure you?"

"No. They wouldn't accept the treatment. They told me, 'You're crazy to treat people that way.' So I had all that responsibility on my own shoulders. I'd say to the patient, 'Now look, I may be able to help you when nothing else has. You've tried everything else. Now try this if you wish.' But that doesn't mean I couldn't have been sued, and I wouldn't have had a Chinaman's chance if something had actually happened.

"Well, my experience is such that I feel very pleased and proud if I wanted to brag about it. What I've done in my lifetime with bees I've been justified in doing. As I look back on it, I am very happy with what I was able to do. I've seen people who just couldn't walk, who are now walking. Those are the things that thrill the hell out of you.

"You know those that failed—what happened? Most of them didn't continue with the treatment. They got too discouraged too soon. Or they'd had arthritis for years and thought they'd get well in a week. People are funny.

"I can truthfully say that I'm satisfied with what I've done over a lifetime. I could've done better, could've done more, but I didn't get any help, any encouragement. My biggest regret was having old Beck die because I could always write to him for help."

"Dr. Carey, I want to thank you and your bride for a very

enjoyable and enlightening visit. I look forward to seeing you again."

"Thank you, son, and good luck with your book."

I had trouble starting the van. I don't know whether I had flooded the carburetor or it was the mist in my head. But I did know that forever more, when I need quiet courage to get me through the day, I remember Dr. Carey.

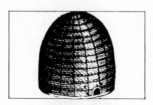

SEVEN

AT THE United States Department of Agriculture bee research lab in Tucson, Arizona, I was given the name of a rheumatologist in New York City who was doing research in bee venom therapy.

I also learned that the late James Hambleton, who for many years was in charge of apiculture research for the USDA in Beltsville, Maryland, used bee stings on arthritics.

It's rather interesting to note that at the same time Mr. Hambleton was treating people with bee stings in the offices of the USDA, Senator Aiken of Vermont asked the Surgeon General to find out if there was anything to the bee venom therapy. His reply to Senator Aiken was, "There is absolutely nothing to it."

In Tucson I met my first beekeeper who had had arthritis for any length of time. Mr. W.J. Lusby had it in two fingers. Mr. Lusby is eighty-six.

"Sometimes it pains me in the middle of the night. I just get up and go out to the hive and put one or two bees on it. They do their work and I go back to sleep."

"How long have you had arthritis?"

"Since I was ten. Had it bad when I was young, but it don't bother much now."

"How long have you been keeping bees?"

"Fifty-six years."

"Maybe that has helped you."

"If I didn't have the bees all these years, I'd probably look like this."

Mr. Lusby assumed the fetal position.

Mrs. Lusby told me that honey cappings are good for the relief of asthma and allergies. The "capping" is the top of the comb, which is sliced off to let the honey drain out. It contains a lot of pollen.

I heard repeatedly that doctors send allergy and asthma patients to get these cappings from beekeepers who operate within ten miles of their homes. If you can't get cappings, chew honeycomb and eat raw honey.

In Dr. Beck's book, *Honey and Health,* we find the following:

Now comes Dr. George D. McGrew, of the Army Medical Corps of the William Beaumont General Hospital in El Paso, Texas, with a statement in an article published in the *Military Surgeon* that during the 1936 hay-fever season thirty-three hay-fever sufferers obtained partial or complete relief through the consumption of honey, produced in their vicinity. The brood cells contain a considerable amount of bee-bread (pollen) stored by the bees for their young and when this is orally administered it will produce a gradual immunity against the allergic symptoms caused by the same pollen. Dr. McGrew found particular relief for patients when they chewed the honey with the wax of the brood cells. The hospital staff also made an alcoholic extract from pollen and administered it in from one to ten drop doses, according to the requirements of the patients.

Mrs. Lusby told me there was a prominent lawyer in town who frequently had to ask for a continuance of his scheduled trials because he suffered so with asthma. Someone put him on to cappings, and he's never had to ask for a continuance since. And he says it's a lot cheaper than an allergist.

Several months later my son Chris had a friend visiting him who was having great trouble breathing because of an asthma attack. I gave him some wildflower honey packaged by Dave McGinnis in Edgewater, Florida, which is some miles from Victoria, British Columbia. He got almost instant relief.

Bumper sticker in Deming, New Mexico: "Have You Hugged Your Kid Today?"

The desert wind was blowing cold and hard when I knocked on J. Ellis's door. I had spent a restless night on the desert among the cactus. The night was clear, but the wind rocked my van. I was impatient and had started to leave when Joe came around from the backyard.

"Sure—be glad to talk bees."

Joe told me that when there is good honey flow in the desert, his hives sometimes increase their weight by twenty-five pounds a day.

Joe told me that whenever he is called to get a swarm of bees, he wears as little clothing as possible—just for effect. He says people always gather around (not too close) and worry out loud that he's going to get stung.

"Honeybees when they swarm have their bellies full of honey and they're just like a man with his belly full—gentle."

I laughed at this because I had long ago told my four kids that if they wanted to persuade a man to do something, ask him after he's just eaten his supper. They practiced what I preached on me.

Joe told me about a fellow beekeeper who used to collect all his dead bees for a woman in Columbus who had rheumatoid arthritis.

"What did she do with them?"

"She put them in a blender, liquefied them, and drank them."

"Oh, my gosh! Did it help?"

"Damned if I know." He said he guessed not, because she didn't get them anymore.

I told Joe about a retirement community I had heard about in Nevada where a small hardware store was selling WD 40, a silicone spray lubricant, by the gross. It seems folks there spray it on the arthritic joints and rub it in.

Well, I guess that's no weirder than bee stings.

An hour or so later I was picking my way up one narrow street and down the next in an old Mexican town called Mesilla.

Joe had advised me to look up a beekeeper named Felipe Garcias. It was a crumbling neighborhood, and with my broken hearing I was not having much success following the directions to Felipe's house.

I said, "The hell with it, I'm going to Texas," and turned up a side street to get back on I-10. There, on this side street, was a neat brick home with a sign modestly proclaiming, "Honey."

Mrs. "Tuffy" Clayshulte answered the door and explained that her husband was the beekeeper, but she would be glad to talk with me.

Mrs. Clayshulte is one of the most poised and erudite women I have met. I felt almost a compulsion to tell her about the peculiar connection between cancer and beekeepers.

She spoke about a symposium she had attended in California and an address given by Dr. Virginia Livingston. Dr. Livingston has a cancer clinic in San Diego, and her success in curing or arresting the disease is 60 percent.

When I left the Clayshultes' they gave me a copy of the address and a two-pound jar of mesquite honey, which soothed and restored this weary traveler.

That night, about 4,000 feet up in the Apache Mountains just west of Boracho, Texas, I found a level spot next to a dry creek. The night air was cold. The moon was full and the stars sparse.

After some wine, cheese, and Campbell's Chunky Turkey Soup, I slipped under my eiderdown to read Dr. Livingston's scientific paper, which Mrs. Clayshulte had given me.

I could almost read by the moonlight coming in through my bubble.

Dr. Livingston said that people who have had tuberculosis or leprosy never get cancer. Hmmm, that's good to know.

Dr. Livingston theorized that we all have a cancer-producing microbe in us. For some undetermined reason, the microbe starts producing hormones, and it is the hormones that are responsible for the explosive cancerous growth. The only way to stop the hormone production is with enzymes.

Interesting.

Sometimes it's a long ride between beekeepers in Texas—597 miles to the next one. Perhaps you'd like to know a little more about the van. You've already noticed that gas station attendants usually go bananas for it and it pulls a lot of eyeballs going down the road.

Well it's a '74 Ford Econoline. I cut a four-by-eight-foot section out of the roof, built a mahogany frame two inches thick and fourteen inches high around the perimeter of the opening, and mounted a four-foot-square smoked Plexiglas bubble on the rear half. In front of that I have a flat sheet of smoked Plexiglas.

I not only get to see the stars, moon, and birds nightly, I also get to see the bottom side of a rain splash, and not many of us can lay claim to that.

My lady, Jeannie MacMillan, gave me the bubble, and I believe it may be on its way to becoming a continental legend.

Over the left rear fender well I have a pantry; and over the right I have a modest library and clothespress. Also on the right side is a refrigerator that operates off the battery, 110 AC, or propane.

It makes a cube or two for an occasional libation or stinging.

On the left side I have shelves halfway up, covered by mahogany panels that lift up parallel with the floor to form two chairs and a table. "Joy," a nude statuette, graces the top of the table shelf. I may very well be in love with her.

The back of the van is given over to a mahogany kitchen counter in which is mounted a two-burner stove, a stainless-steel sink, and a cutting board I made from part of Bill Darrid's old diving board. This may be a safer use of it. Over the sink is a removable five-gallon water reservoir.

In an alcove over the sink I have mounted an old bell given me by Fleurette Martin (one of my rose ladies) on the occasion of my launching the caique *Oremus*. This green corroded brass beauty is about 300 years old and was retrieved from a sunken Spanish vessel near Key Largo.

Rolled up underneath the kitchen counter is a foam rubber mattress that serves me comfortably when unrolled. For warmth I have an eiderdown quilt with an exquisite patchwork coverlet made by my daughter Kathy.

Mounted on the mahogany roof frame is a ship's clock with proper bells and a matching barometer. The bells sound every half hour in four-hour sequences and tickle hell out of me every time I hear them. Also on this frame is a haunting photo of the Oregon coastline given to me by Merlene Brennand, a special friend.

Mounted over the engine in a mahogany housing, polished to a high gloss, is an FM radio and tape deck and a lighted brass compass. There are several holes for glasses or cups, and a storage compartment.

From side to side and over the windshield is a shelf containing all manner of tapes. In fact, sufficient tapes to take me across the country and back and never repeat a selection. Benny Goodman, Bechet, Bluegrass, Beethoven, Leon Redbone, Carly Simon, Carole King, John Denver, Neil Diamond, Peggy Lee, Willie Dixon, etc. I like most music of the Western world except I get a little squirrely on chamber music. Perhaps I've been in the wrong chambers.

And mounted up on the dash, always in view, I have a tiny bluebird of happiness given me by Lois Copping, my daughter Judi's mother-in-law. And it works.

Some people say the van reminds them of a yacht. This is not happenstance. I designed it so. I really wanted to build a thirty-five-foot ketch, but the realities of economics deemed otherwise.

I couldn't be more pleased with the van. I can tuck it away on an old logging road, sneak down by the ocean, hobnob with cows, and get a freebie sandwiched between GM extravaganzas in a Holiday Inn parking lot. And I always sleep under the stars, raindrops, or snowflakes.

Saturday morning I pulled into Paris, Texas, to see Mr. Meier, the manager of Dadant's Beekeeping Supply Store. His son explained that his dad was away for the weekend, but that he would talk to me if I wanted to wait until he finished with his customers.

The lad was only about nineteen or twenty, and I thought he would not be heavily steeped in bee lore. But I hadn't talked with anyone for a day or so and perhaps I was a little lonely. I waited.

Well, I'll be darned. This lad had been to the Mayo Clinic to cure his allergy to bee venom because he wanted to follow his father in the bee business. After a series of injections with bee venom serum in Rochester, he was deemed not allergic to bee stings. However, in order to maintain this immunity he must give himself the sting every two weeks. If he misses these booster shots, he may have to go through the entire series of injections again.

The attending physician had permitted him to watch while he treated a woman with arthritis of the knee by injecting *bee venom serum.*

I also learned that some Mexican beemen had donated five pounds of royal jelly to a group of American scientists who were doing research on cancer. The boy didn't know how they were using it.

But perhaps most important of all, young Mr. Meier gave me some back editions of the *American Bee Journal.*

Heading northwest from Paris, I was following a slow-moving line of traffic, skipping back and forth across the median line looking for an opportunity to pass. I suddenly realized that all the opposing traffic had pulled off onto the shoulder. Hell, I thought, that sure is accommodating. Now I can make my pass. But I delayed just a bit, for I had never before experienced this sort of behavior from oncoming traffic.

It's good I did hesitate because at the end of that hesitation the line in front of me turned right—into a cemetery. Up north we slow down a bit when an oncoming funeral procession approaches, but this pulling off the road was something else again.

I sometimes think we make too much of dying.

For years my family has had precise instructions from me. No funeral, no wake, and the night they slip me in the ground I want a gangbuster party. Lots of old Benny Goodman records, foods both plentiful and exciting, and lots of booze.

I have my epitaph picked out. I ordered it chiseled on a five-foot slab of Vermont granite. I canceled the order when I learned that the stone would weigh 500 or 600 pounds and that I would be on the road, rambling about for the next several years.

Nothing fancy. Just:

HERE LIES FRED
DEAD

Whenever I recited this epitaph at a party, my wife invariably would add:

[WE HOPE]

Which invariably evoked the response, "Oh, Lynne, you have such a good sense of humor." To which she invariably responded, "I have to have in order to stay married to Fred."

But I guess she lost it.

That night I poked around in the innards of the Ozarks looking for a safe harbor. It was dusk, and in the dim light the nearby railroad tracks looked rusty. That was fine. I'd have a quiet night with the stars ticking down, if the coon hunters didn't eat me.

I picked up the January 1972 edition of the *American Bee Journal* young Meier had given me and read an article by the pharmacologist James A. Vick in which he describes the fractionation of bee venom. The eighth component is *enzymes.*

Hot damn, *enzymes!* Just what Dr. Livingston had mentioned.

The old scalp started tingling unlike it had since the time I was nineteen and OD'd on Vicks nosedrops. I mean I could hardly contain myself.

What with that and six or seven freight trains highballing through my living room all night, I didn't sleep much.

Is this, then, the reason for the low incidence of cancer in beekeepers?

Joe Parkhill of Berryville, Arkansas, told me an interesting tale. The federal government sent three scientists to Brazil to see what could be done about preventing the Africanized Brazilian bee from becoming ensconced in the United States.

They spent $300,000 and came back with no answers.

Joe made a long-distance phone call to Dr. Eva Crane, one of the world's leading authorities on bees, and for $8 got the answer.

Dr. Crane said, "Don't worry about those bees, Joe, they don't cluster."

Bees must cluster (huddle together for warmth) in temperate climates, even Florida, in order to survive in cool weather.

It's a pity the $300,000 was not spent on bee venom or honey research.

During the course of the winter, Joan Smith, the statuesque Tennessee redhead, had written to 155 doctors throughout the United States and Europe who practice preventive medicine. The essence of the query was: "Do you use bee venom in treating arthritis and/or do you know anyone who does?" Eighty-one of the doctors were kind enough to respond:

Don't know anything about it	45
Would like to know about it	9
Know it has been or is being used	22
Use it on patients	5

Here are some excerpts from those who know bee venom is being used for arthritis therapy:

Casper, Wyoming
I believe this approach does have merit and that in the future it may be proven to be of great benefit.

Southfield, Mississippi

Have no information on this, though persons accidently stung by bees have sometimes reported such relief. There is always danger of allergic shock reaction.

Far Rockaway, New York

Yes, I've heard of the treatment and I know it's being used extensively in Europe. Unfortunately, I know of no sources or information on applicability. I just know it works as a counterirritant and removes toxic acids from the stiffened joint. If you get any information from other sources, I'd appreciate knowing about it.

Lowville, New York

I am only acquainted with the fact that bee sting is effective in treating arthritis and have had no experience with such treatment. Best wishes and good luck!

Quebec, Canada

I do have some patients who have used self-administered bee stings for arthritis, with remarkable results. As far as bee venom, and where to secure this, I cannot be of any assistance.

Kalamazoo, Michigan

I have been well aware of the fact that bee venom is effective with arthritic cases. I would be interested to find out what you learn in your research.

Covina, California

Any allergist can give you these injections. I've known of a few patients who've responded.

Some excerpts from doctors who use it:

Riehen, Switzerland

We have worked with bee venom in cases of arthritis and this treatment was successful. We took bee venom in middle potencies, as D6 and D12.

Göttingen, West Germany

We use bee venom in different forms in Germany. For instance, in a homeopathic form as Apis D3 or in combination with other homeopathic ingredients in Arthribosan, produced by Walter Bock Gmbh & Co. KG, Hellkampstr. 7, Postfach 305, D4650 Gelsenkirchen

—or in the form of injections, ointments or liniments called: Forapin ampullen, Forapin salbe, Forapin liniment, produced by Heinrich Mack Nachfolger, Chemisch-Pharmazuetische Fabrik, Postfach 140, D-7918 Illertissen/Bayern. Please ask the producers for exact information. I hope I could help you.

Somewhere in Alabama

I am sorry, but I don't have any information of any other doctors using this as a treatment. I use it myself as a treatment, but do not know any other one who is doing it. I have had very good results with it and it does seem to help. I have been using this therapy for ten to twelve years intermittently. It works really well on rheumatoid arthritis and perhaps even better on osteoarthritis.

I have treated over 100 people. About 25 percent recovered completely; 40 percent showed great improvement; 20 percent showed some improvement. There were none in which the condition worsened. The only side effects—one patient developed a skin rash at the site of injection and this responded well to medication. Several days later venom treatment was resumed and the rash did not reappear.

I have not published anything about this therapy—have been hesitant to do so because of the FDA.

Westland, Mississippi

Work best with Verniton injector—small doses at site of pain.

Orlando, Florida

Thank you for your letter regarding bee venom. This is a modality of great importance, but it's been ten or fifteen years since I've done this procedure and at the present time I do not know who supplies the venom. It is outlawed by the medical profession and it is hard to find. It could be that a search will have to be made in Europe to get the material. If I find any information on this, I will let you know.

Curious how commonplace this therapy is in Europe and how timid American medicine is about investigating the possibilities.

I detoured 300 miles to see a friend who is a pharmacist, hoping to excite him with my tales of honey and bee venom.

"If this stuff's so damn good, why don't we know about it?" he said.

Indeed.

The following is reprinted in part from the *American Bee Journal,* January 1977. Dr. F.B. Wells, a chemist:

In 1933, without warning, a partially crippling condition developed suddenly in the left ankle and . . . for years often interfered seriously with walking. Although several treatments were prescribed by different doctors and followed carefully for considerable periods of time, none gave any apparent relief. Then, in 1942 I took up beekeeping in the back yard. An occasional sting was experienced without any apparent effect on the ankle until late one afternoon, while walking near a couple of hives, there was a sting right on the sorest spot of the ankle. Within a half hour the ankle was so swollen and so hot that it was not only almost immobilized, but it seemed the skin must surely burst, become crisp, or both. After two days, swelling and temperature had both subsided somewhat but these inconveniences were then replaced with an itch that surely could never be surpassed. At the end of a week the ankle was in good condition and to this day there has been no recurrence of inflammation or irritation of any kind. The ankle is never a consideration in cases of walks regardless of length or terrain.

I have presented my case to several doctors along with the question of why they do not even consider bee sting therapy. You wouldn't believe the excuses and evasions by men who supposedly believe their Hippocratic Oath, and who supposedly have the interests of their patients at heart. To illustrate, I present a representative composite, and I stress, composite, question and answer series based, to the best of my memory, on the most common replies by doctors.

Q. *Based on my experience I am moved to ask why do you not advocate use of bee sting therapy in the treatment of arthritic conditions.*

A. It cannot possibly be done under antiseptic conditions at the present time and, besides, patients would not stand for being stung.

Q. *But sterile venom is available for use by injection just like other drugs and compositions; and by its use the patient need never fear the sting. So, why not use it?*

A. Its use could be dangerous. Some people are allergic to bee stings.

Q. *You do not object to but often even suggest allergy tests for other things so why balk at such tests for bee venom?*

A. Well, one cannot be assured of results even if the allergy tests are negative.

Q. *There are many other treatments for which you cannot guarantee results, but since some have had success with them you do not hesitate to try them. Why not try this one?*

A. There is not enough clinical evidence available.

Q. *Why not make your own clinical evidence starting with my case? All clinical evidence had to start with the first treatment somewhere. If all treatment had to be based on previous clinical evidence we would have absolutely no usable treatments today.*

A. I did not treat you so you are not evidence at all.

This could go on indefinitely but by now a certain degree of irritation usually becomes apparent as does the very obvious fact that bee venom treatment is "out."

Yes, indeed.

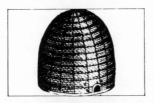

EIGHT

I WAS heading south on Alabama Highway 431 when I entered Lafayette. Weathered pine board shacks lined 431 on the north end of town. No paint, no glass in the windows, barely supported by four cement blocks. I imagined it looked much like the set for *The Grapes of Wrath*. There were some folks sitting on the porches and on the steps. They didn't look depressed. But depression enveloped me like hot air swishing from an eighteen-wheeler in the Mojave Desert.

The center of Lafayette is pretty much like a hundred other southern and western towns of 3,500. A square with the town offices in the center; a movie house, furniture store, and diner; some people eyeballed my bubble and my mahogany.

However, the southern end of the town is something else: high lawns with beautifully designed homes and well-executed landscaping. The affluence at this end of town nearly ran down the gutters.

I don't understand how you can live this way without your conscience gnawing at you. But obviously we learn how. The Puritan ethic doubtless is a comfort.

My next stop was Auburn. I checked the phone book for Dr.

Guyton. There was a Guyton—in fact seven of them, and none listed as doctor. Would you believe the first one I dialed was *the* Dr. Guyton? It was raining so he couldn't tend his camelias. Yes, he could talk with me.

"You know how I got into this thing? Of course, I taught bee culture for forty-two years at the university, and almost always somebody in the class would say, 'Well, professor, I hear that bee stings will cure arthritis.'

"I knew Beck had had his book out, and somebody asked about it one day. I guess I must have smiled because the boy spoke up and said, 'Professor, you don't need to smile.' I said, 'Why?' He said, 'Cause it'll do it.'

"I said, 'Jack, how do you know?'

"He said his college doctor had sent him home with arthritis of his upper extremities to such an extent that he couldn't stay in college and the doctors couldn't do anything for him.

"His pain became so terrific that he stripped to his waist and went out in front of an old beehive and took a stick and poked in, and they got him thirty-eight times before he got away.

"I said, 'Jack, don't you know that might have killed you?' He said, 'It didn't matter. My pain was so severe I'd just as soon have died as not.' He was back in school in one week. He lives down the road here. He's just retired as county agent. He's never had another attack of arthritis. His name is Jack Bolden.

"I had it in my right knee shortly after that. I just had occasional sharp pain in my knee, but I couldn't take a full step. When I got into a car, I had to pick my leg up and put it in, and when I'd get out, I'd pick the leg up and put it out. I said, 'Well, I'll try Jack's cure.' I pulled up my pants leg and put five stings on my right knee. In a couple of days the pain was gone, just like that. Had arthritis in my wrist. Did the same thing on my wrist and it cleared up.

"Had an old gentleman from a neighboring city. He was the worst case I ever saw. I tell you, my heart fell when I saw him —his wristwatch was embedded right in his wrist. They had to carry him into the office.

"He looked up and said, 'Professor what can you do for me?' That was hard to answer. I said, 'Mr. Levin, I have great faith and I've seen miraculous results—at least we'll try. Where's your worst place?'

" 'My neck, if I can't get relief in my neck I'm going to kill myself.'

"His wife had to minister to him all through the night with hot towels and so forth, and in three weeks we got him up to where he had complete use of himself, drove his truck, and went about his business.

"He got some bees and treated himself after that.

"A lot of these things, Mr. Malone, make me wonder: Is it all in the head? Is arthritis all in the head? I don't know.

"I had an old gentleman from near Birmingham. He was sixty-three years old. Best bone man in the state had him in metal braces from his shoulders to his hips. He came down. I treated him. I said, 'Mr. Smith, I want to know the very worst spot you have. I want to treat it first. And if you stay overnight and you've had no bad reaction, I'll treat you again in the morning before you go home.'

"He said, 'Professor, that left hip hasn't been without pain for twenty-five years.' So I put one sting on his left hip. I met him in the doctor's office the next morning at eight o'clock, and I said, 'How are you feeling, Mr. Smith?' He said, 'Professor, I expect you'll think I'm crazy. I haven't had a pain in that hip since you put that sting on me.'

"Well, I thought he was crazy. That kind of thing, is it in the head? Is it? It makes me wonder."

"But you must have had a lot of people come to you with a great deal of skepticism in their minds. And they were helped."

"Oh, yes, they came with skepticism and fear of the sting and in a short time they'd be yelling 'put 'em here, put 'em there.' "

I think it's worthwhile to interrupt Professor Guyton here for just a moment. The question of "is it all in the head" comes up every time I get into my bee venom/arthritis tales. However, the following are two pieces of evidence that I think indicate that it is not basically "in the head."

Research Communications in Chemical Pathology and Pharmacology, September 1972, printed an article titled, "Influence of Bee Venom in the Adjuvant-Induced Arthritic Rat Model," by G.J. Lorenzetti, B. Fortenberry, and E. Busby of Alcan Laboratories, Fort Worth, Texas:

> The adjuvant-induced arthritic rat model was utilized for evaluating the anti-inflammatory activity of bee venom. Administration of bee venom subcutaneously was found to prevent the arthritic syndromes in this animal model when the compound was administered therapeutically and prophylactically. The anti-inflammatory effect was more pronounced in the prophylactic regimen. Results indicate that bee venom should be investigated further for its possible anti-arthritic activity.

In February 1975, James A. Vick, Glenn B. Warren, and Robert Brooks published "The Effect of Treatment with Whole Bee Venom on Daily Cage Activity and Plasma Cortisol Levels in the Arthritic Dog":

> Whole bee venom increases daily cage activity in dogs with arthritis. It is also apparent from these studies that venom is effective only when injections are given over a prolonged period of time. That is, the arthritic dogs in Group III showed some decrease in cage activity within 30 days after discontinuance of the bee venom injections. However, none of the four arthritic dogs returned to their pretreatment cage activity levels even when the plasma cortisol levels returned to normal.
>
> It appears from these studies that injections of whole bee venom stimulate both the production of cortisol and the average daily cage activity of arthritic dogs. Whole bee venom does not appear to increase activity levels in dogs which do not show arthritic signs nor does saline injection into arthritic dogs produce any increase in their cage activity.

The above article was published in the *American Bee Journal.* The authors could find no scientific journal publisher in the United States who would print it. It was finally published in an English scientific journal. Those of you who cling to the notion that the profession is intractable in its pursuit of medical truth, are you sure?

Now back to the professor.

"It got so they almost liked to be stung, is that right?" I asked.

"Oh, I had one woman I treated for three or four years. And I did everything in the world I knew to get rid of her. I'd say, 'Let's skip it for a week, let's skip it for two weeks.' She'd skip, and then she'd be right back, right back. That old lady had to walk to the office, and she said she just couldn't get along without them.

"So the next thing that comes to mind is, 'Is bee sting habit forming?' Couldn't be anything like that."

"I don't know. Broadman and also Beck felt there was some narcotic substance to it," I said.

"I treated between 1942 and 1956 and I was very fortunate. This was before the age of suing for everything. I had to get out of it because I had a heavy load and I was afraid of losing everything I've got through some crooked lawyer. My doctor didn't want me to quit.

"Had a lady from New Orleans, a Mrs. Knight, who wrote me and had written to Purdue University to get information on bee venom. They referred her to Baton Rouge Bee Laboratory, and of course Baton Rouge referred her to me. We got in correspondence and I gave her recommendations for treatment and so forth.

"She had been to Oschner Clinic, and they had told her there was absolutely no help for her."

"Where is that clinic, Professor?"

"New Orleans. That's the famous clinic in New Orleans. She started taking bee sting treatments and one day, when I was over at the office, the phone rang and it was Mrs. Knight.

" 'How are you, Mrs. Knight? Where are you?' She said she was in Auburn. She's bedfast, remember, completely bedfast. 'I'm in Auburn,' she said, 'and I want to come over and see you.'

"I was on the third floor and I wanted to meet her downstairs in the parking lot because the stairs were so hard. By the time I finished with my class and started down the hall, here came Mrs. Knight on the third floor. Bedfast case, her husband had administered the bees to her, and there she was in Auburn after the Oschner Clinic had said there was no hope for her. It's amazing. It's amazing.

"There's no question in my mind that it is the most efficacious treatment for arthritis that has ever been used."

"Why don't doctors use it?" I asked.

"Well, they haven't had experience with handling bees. They have not had any experience with it. Carey was a medical man, and he knew how to handle bees. My brother lived out in California and I had him go by to appraise Carey for me. He had a visit with Carey and gave him a very, very fine recommendation. I had correspondence with Dr. Carey, and all the advice he gave me was good. He said never give up on a case in less than six months.

"I had a young man who had very severe pain in his shoulder, and I didn't get any result with him for six months. About the end of six months he started to get relief. Then it looked like every week we gained on it, until we completely wiped it out. I've seen him not too long ago. He's county agent and he's never had a recurrence.

"But they do have recurrences. No use getting the idea it won't come back after you've cleared it up with bee stings."

I asked Professor Guyton if it always came back.

"No, no, it doesn't always come back. I had a number of cases where it never came back. But I've had them where it did come back."

"What would you say your rate of success was, Professor?"

"I treated over 100 cases and I think I helped all but maybe five or six. One of those had venereal origins and several more became sensitized and we had to quit.

"I desensitized one woman, a Mrs. Wilson. I gave her one sting for one minute and she reacted pretty seriously to it. Then I started putting the sting on for just a few seconds, increased gradually. Finally got to where I could give her thirty-five or forty stings at a time. Never had any bad results."

"Did you ever treat bursitis?"

"One case. My wife had bursitis. The doctor told her he was probably going to have to go in there with a needle and wash the calcium out. I said, 'Let's try the bees first.' In two or three treatments it was gone. It cleared up. She never had it anymore.

"I had a professor who ran a thorn in this finger joint and the joint swelled up like a balloon. His doctor treated it and treated it and finally told him he couldn't do him any good. So the professor asked me if I would treat it, and I said, 'Only in your doctor's office. I won't treat it anywhere else.' And so his doctor gave him permission—he didn't believe in this bee business.

"I don't know how many times I treated him—four, five, or six weeks—something like that. Cleared it out completely—normal, all the swelling gone. I called his doctor in and said, 'Doctor, I would like you to examine this now.' He stood off ten feet and said, 'Well you did cure one didn't you?'

"We had a doctor here who gave venom hypodermically. He called me in finally and asked me to give his patients some live bee stings.

"One old man had high blood pressure. Dr. Terc claimed that following bee sting therapy high blood pressure or low blood pressure tended to reach normalcy. This man had high blood pressure, and since he had had hypodermic injections before by the doctor, my first treatment was six stings in the back. His blood pressure started coming down.

"I said, 'Doctor his blood pressure is down. You want to blame that on the bee stings?' 'Oh, no,' he says, 'I'm treating him for that.' But he could not get rid of his arthritis with the bee venom serum. I treated him half a dozen times with live bees. Cleared it right up.

"It was a marvelous experience for me, a marvelous experience. I wouldn't go through it again for anybody. But my compensation—I'd never take any money for it, never took anything except I think I got a camelia plant one time and a turkey one time for Christmas dinner—the compensation was terrific."

"I would think so."

"No money could take the place of that. But I wouldn't do it again. I couldn't afford to take the risk. They sue you now at the drop of a hat."

Somehow I didn't believe Dr. Guyton would refuse to do it again. Even with the risk involved.

I reviewed the professor's notes that night and Sunday morning. When I returned the notes he told me to be sure and look up a former student of his, Professor Frank Robinson, at the University of Florida. It was a pleasure being with Dr. Guyton, and I hope to visit with him again someday.

On the outskirts of town I picked up a young couple, Terri Davis and Richard Sink. They were hitchhiking from West Virginia to Panama City, Florida. They slept under trees by the side of the road, which is far braver than sleeping in a van. And wouldn't you know it, the girl kept bees. When they left they said they liked my van, they liked my music, and they liked my company. Nice folks.

The only other hitchhiker I picked up in all my travels was Max Leader. Max is about sixty and very bright. He was just north of Ascutney, Vermont. Max always hitches in a bulging business suit and full beard. Max (actually his name is Herb, but I'll always think of him as Max) looked over my van and said, "Here's a motto for you."

He handed me a crumpled State of Vermont officer's citation for hitchhiking. On the back he had scratched *"Omnia Mea Mecum Porto,"* which means everything I own I carry with me. Boy, was I impressed! I took three years of Latin and all I can write is *Dominus vobiscum.*

I told him I was going to write a book on bee venom as a cure for arthritis.

"I used to have bees," he said. "Had twenty-five hives once. That's bullshit."

"Do you have arthritis?" I asked.

"No."

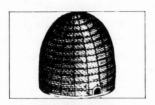

NINE

PROFESSOR FRANK ROBINSON, entomologist at the University of Florida, introduced me to two products he had brought back from Germany.

Mack, a German drug firm, produces an injectable bee venom serum, Forapin, and a bee venom ointment that is widely used in Europe. Mack maintains over 1,300 hives in West Germany just for venom. It is the largest apiarist in the country.

I smeared a little ointment on my left index finger. For the first hour or so it felt like Vaseline. But after that the finger became very red and burned considerably. This is a good sign. The Germans hold Forapin ointment in high regard, Mr. Robinson said.

Happily, Pfizer has bought 95 percent ownership of Mack, so maybe, just maybe, someday Americans too will have benefits from the serum and ointment.

The countryside around Umatilla is—well, almost delicious. The orange groves were in bloom and the sun warm. Actually, the sun was hot.

"Is the sun bothering you, Mr. Brew?"

"Yes, it is. Let's get under this orange tree. I'll never forget the opening. Almost the first sentence of that account of the works from France on royal jelly was: 'The most notable characteristic of royal jelly is that it stimulates the action of every gland in your body.' They even made spayed white rats come into heat."

"Do you take royal jelly, Mr. Brew?"

"Every time I find some queen cells, I eat me a little royal jelly. I wish I would eat it more often. I do that about like I do everything else. I start out to do it about like keeping my books —for a couple of weeks I'll do it, and after that I'll find a way to get out of it.

"But the truth is almost no one does anything unless they sense a demand from something, and a fellow who really feels good is not going to make much effort to do anything."

There are a number of stories I can relate that attest to the power of honey to cure ulcers. I favor Mr. Brew's story.

"When I was eighteen years old I got a job with the State of New York inspecting bees. One Sunday afternoon I was fixing to leave home because I had to go a long way to work and I was visiting with my mother.

"I asked my mother how was Earl Pobacker. I hadn't seen him for a month. 'Oh, my,' she says, 'Earl is terrible, in bed. He's almost invalid with ulcers.' It really made me sad because he was like a second father to me, wonderful old guy. So I said, 'Well I'm going to stop and see him before I pull out of here. Remembering all those buckets of honey he bought from me years ago, I'm going to take him one.'

"So I walked into his bedroom after greeting his wife. It hit me. You know at that age back in the country in them Depression days, I don't think I had ever seen but one or two dead people, and that man, so different from what he had been and in that bed, looked like a ghost to me; he almost looked like a corpse. Affected me terribly, although I tried not to let him see it.

"I let a little time go by till I could get my composure and had as good a little visit with him as I could.

"With the idea of leaving, I told him I had brought him a bucket of honey. He thanked me for it, but said his doctors wouldn't allow him to eat it. All he could eat was some baby food and sweet cream and stuff like that.

"I said, 'Well now, Earl, just looking at you I wouldn't say them doctors are doing too good by you, and I can assure you that I have read books written by medical doctors who absolutely recommend honey for ulcers, and it makes good sense to me.'

"And I said, 'You've got a good system. It's just that you're starved to death. Your stomach ain't giving you any food. Just dip the spoon in the honey and lick the spoon a little. Just get a few drops into you, then wait thirty minutes and if you don't have any gastric pains try a few more drops.'

"When I got home the next week I found out that he had got up out of bed and gone over home to thank my mother and father, and he got over his ulcers."

N. Ioyrish, in *Bees and People,* says:

In the period 1944–9, 600 patients with ulcers of the stomach were treated with honey at the clinic of the Irkutsk [Soviet Union] Medical Institute. M.L. Khotkina (1953) described 221 cases with the most typical course: 76 (34.3 per cent) had hyperacidity; 67 (30.2 per cent) were normal; in 54 (24.7 per cent) acidity was subnormal; and in 24 (10.8 per cent) there was no acidity. When the normal diet and medicines were prescribed 61 per cent of the patients recovered and 18 per cent still felt pain; but when honey was prescribed 79.7 to 84.3 per cent recovered and only 5.9 continued to feel pain at the end of treatment. X-ray established that, with normal treatment, the ulcers healed in 29 per cent of patients, but in 59.2 per cent of those taking honey. The average period of hospitalization was shorter for patients prescribed honey. A general tonic effect was also noted: weight increased, the composition of the blood improved, gastric acidity became normal, and there was a tranquillizing effect on the nervous system. Patients became calm, cheerful, and full of life.

For ulcers honey should be taken 90 minutes to two hours before meals, or three hours afterward, preferably an hour and a half or two hours before breakfast and the midday meal and three hours after the evening meal. The honey should be dissolved in warm, boiled water.

In this form it dilutes the mucus in the stomach and lowers acidity, and is rapidly assimilated without irritating the intestine. A cold solution, on the other hand, increases acidity, slows down digestion of the contents of the stomach, and irritates the intestine. When taken just before meals, honey stimulates secretion of gastric juice.

In 1938, Dr. Beck wrote in *Honey and Health:*

Dr. Schacht, of Wiesbaden, claims to have cured many hopeless cases of gastric and intestinal ulcers with honey and without operations. It is rather unusual that a physician of standing has the courage and conviction to praise honey. The beekeepers and their friends know that honey will cure gastric and intestinal ulcerations, this distressing, prevalent and most dangerous malady, a precursor of cancer. But the news has not yet reached 99% of the medical profession. The remaining few physicians who know it, are afraid to suggest such an unscientific and plebeian remedy, for fear of being laughed at by their colleagues.

Mr. Arthur Brew's grammar was a little ragged, but he is a learned man with many deep thoughts and clear concepts. I enjoyed visiting with him, but I had to leave the shade of the orange tree and git.

There were days of disappointments doing research for this book. Difficulties locating the beekeepers, who were usually out in the country; finding beekeepers who knew less than I did; and so forth. But, like selling, you have your ups and downs, and success was just a matter of making the calls.

One afternoon I was in a blue funk because I seemed to be on a long down cycle. I knocked on the door of Rossie Hambrick's mobile home. She lives alone and was a little worried about me until she learned I wanted to talk bees.

Mrs. Hambrick had a serious accident in 1960 and "after that arthritis set in. You see, that knuckle is still not pretty. And that one, when I get up in the morning it's cocked that way and I have to pull it this way. The pain in my arm, in my knee, then around through my rib cage, it was just like a vise being tightened and I was going crazy.

"So I got out there and started playing with the bees. Somebody said, 'It'll take care of it.' I got over 200 stings at one time, and I haven't had arthritis since. It got rid of it; it got rid of it."

"When was that, in 1960?"

"No, in 1962 I got all those stings. I never got arthritis again. That's why you see these bees out here."

"I think they do a lot of good things for us."

"I know it. You see, my husband died—it'll be twenty years the thirteenth of May. I started playing with honeybees instead of playing with men."

I laughed.

"Laugh at me. There's sense in that. I found too many men that want to do just what you're doing right now."

"You mean sit here?"

"Yes, just sit there and let a woman wait on them, and no part of that I'll have."

"We do like to do that."

"Yeah, especially these older men. They're looking for a woman who's got a dollar put away—they want that—and then they want to sit down and tell her monkey jump here, monkey jump there, monkey jump somewhere else. I'd rather go out there and play with the bees."

"Do you take a little royal jelly now and again?"

"I have, yes. I was awfully run down. I had gone from 210 down to 153 pounds, skinny as a rail. This doctor was riding down to the meeting with me one night, and I asked him if he thought it would do me any good to eat some royal jelly. He sat there a while and he looked at me and he said, 'Your husband is dead isn't he? I wouldn't advise you to eat any.' So I guess you know what he meant by that. I'm not so dense that I couldn't figure it out. I dropped the subject right there."

This reminded me of an interview I had had back in northeastern Texas. All across the country I had been asking beekeepers if they used royal jelly. Royal jelly is manufactured by glands in a worker bee's head. It is fed to the larvae in the early stages of their development. If a larva is fed exclusively on royal jelly, that larva becomes a queen, which is roughly two and a half times the size and weight of a worker bee. It is powerful stuff in beeland. Fresh royal jelly contains vitamins B_1, B_2, B_6, C; niacin; biotin; inositol; folic acid; and pantothenic acid.

A fair number of old-time beekeepers told me that they took some now and again and it seemed to relax them. Homer Park in California told me that if he took too much he felt like taking a little snooze. I repeated this story to a beeman in Waxahachie, Texas. He had been in the bee business a long time. He was about fifty-five, and his eyes sparkled a mite when I told him the earlier answers I had heard about royal jelly.

"I don't know about that, but when I was a young man, about twenty-one, I'd say, I worked for an old-time bee inspector. He kept telling me about the virtues of royal jelly. Finally, one day I took some. And that night I had an erection that wouldn't quit."

I smiled.

And he smiled just a whisker and said, "Perhaps I better try it again."

In *Bees and People* we find:

Experiments have shown that the life span of animals fed very small amounts of royal jelly is increased by a third. It causes pullets to lay more eggs and stimulates old fowls to begin laying again.

Henry Hale demonstrated in 1939 that royal jelly contains a gonadotropic hormone. Female rats given subcutaneous injections of an extract of the jelly put on weight and exhibited increased follicular activity of the ovaries within a few days.

I drove south on Route A1A through West Palm Beach to Fort Lauderdale—a beautiful drive. I was flabbergasted at the wealth represented by the posh seaside mansions. I wondered how many of these owners were doing something creative.

Fort Lauderdale and I were introduced at the beginning of the spring college recess. Young drivers choked the highway and lean brown bodies crowded the sidewalks. Everything seemed in order at 9 P.M. Most folks looked mildly bored and waiting for a happening. I saw one group point at me and shout, "Hey look at the goddam yacht!" I managed to slip in between a couple of gargantuan motor homes in the Sheraton parking lot to catch a couple of Zs. The night forces restored me. Aside from some loud beer talk periodically, I slept well.

It's funny. The picture my mind conjured up when Florida was mentioned was hundreds of hotels pushing onto the sands of Miami Beach.

And, of course, geographically speaking, Miami Beach is an infinitesimal part of Florida. I was constantly surprised by the number of beautiful lakes down through central Florida. I was delighted by the remote beauty on the Gulf Coast around Cedar Key and the rural detachment of the Panhandle.

I mention this because one morning I drove into Miami Beach for some bacon, eggs, and home fries. Rusting air conditioners hung out of every hotel window, soiling the stucco beneath. I had the feeling Miami Beach was in the throes of receivership. It's a shame that such a pretty state has such a lousy stereotype. I skipped breakfast that morning and got the hell out of Miami Beach.

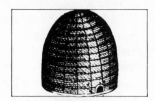

TEN

MRS. HAMBRICK had directed me to Mr. and Mrs. Dick McCoy.

"My doctor will tell you when I went to see him I was crawling. He weren't doing me no good, giving me that cortisone, and it kept getting worse instead of better.

"I come home and told my husband, 'Go get some bees and put some on there.' I hadn't been able to scrub my floor for a week and a half. I let that stinger stay in for twenty minutes, and in thirty minutes I was up scrubbing my kitchen floor.

"When I went back to the doctor for my health card, he said, 'Mrs. McCoy what happened to you? Last time I saw you, you were crawling, just about.' I said, 'Well you're not going to believe this, but I got bee stings.' He said, 'Where did you hear tell of bee stings?'

"I said, 'All my life I've knowed about bee stings.' He said, 'We doctors do what we can. We don't know nothing to do for it, but we try.' And I ain't been back to him since for arthritis."

"I had a heart attack," said Mr. McCoy, "and honey is good for heart patients. So I told her to bring it over by the gallon.

The nurses and doctors and everybody else was wanting honey, but I had my jug of honey there all the time while I was in the hospital.

"I got out of the hospital quicker, the doctors released me faster than what they usually do and told me not to do anything, just rest. It got pretty boring and I was feeling pretty good and I was walking quite a ways. Every day I'd walk. So my doctor sent me back to work earlier than usual, and I kept taking my honey for energy and also for my heart. My doctor bought a case of honey from me after that.

In Ioyrish's *Curative Properties of Honey and Bee Venom,* we find the following:

Since honey consists for the most part of glucose, its beneficial action on the cardiac muscle is quite understandable.

According to some authors (Professor M. B. Goloms, A. Raff and others), the daily consumption [of] from 50 to 140 (an average of 70) grammes of honey for one or two months by patients with serious heart diseases brings about a marked improvement in their condition, normalizes their blood composition, increases the haemoglobin content and the cardiovascular tonus.

Honey was included in the diet of some patients suffering from various diseases with signs of cardiovascular insufficiency; this provided optimal conditions for the nutrition of the myocardium.

Honey should be included in the everyday diet of patients with heart weakness.

During the International Symposium on Apitherapy held in Madrid in 1974, S. Mladenov of Bulgaria stated:

In the case of heart diseases (myocarditis, sthenocarditis and hypertony) treatment with honey contributes to the irrigation of the heart muscles and of its vessels, dilates the blood vessels, improves the irregular heart activity and has a hypotensive effect.

"Migraine headaches. I used to get migraine headaches that lasted for a week," Mr. McCoy said. "A couple of times I've been setting down and felt one coming on. Right away I'd get up and take a couple of tablespoons of honey, lay down or be quiet, calm down, and relax. I have warded off migraine headaches with honey."

The dog barked in the bedroom.

Mrs. McCoy said, "I even give my dog honey. And our vet says the reason she's never had worms is because she eats honey."

Mr. McCoy said, "She's never been wormed. She's never had any worms. When she was a puppy we put honey in her milk. She won't eat her Gainesburgers without honey on it."

I had to tell them about Mrs. Randall telling me she sold honey to the dog track for the greyhounds, just to show I knew something.

Then Mr. McCoy parried with: "The horse tracks use honey," and I knew I was out of my class.

I had missed breakfast this day, but I surely did have a good visit with Mr. and Mrs. McCoy, and I hope they know how much I enjoyed chatting with them.

Bumper sticker in Lakeland: "Car OK—Driver Needs Body Work."

I slipped down to Key Largo to spend some time at the much-heralded John Pennekamp Coral Reef State Park. Fortunately, it was booked ahead for the next several months. I snuck in to replenish my water supply and found the campsites to be exceptionally dusty and crowded close together. This was contrary to every other state park I visited in Florida.

Poking around on the northern tip of Key Largo, I discovered an abandoned asphalt road running along the shoreline. It ran parallel to the traveled road with approximately 100 feet of scrub pine in between. This was more my style.

The ocean moved gently on what I thought was sand, but I soon realized it was ground-down coral. Truly, in two steps I could be from my van into the Atlantic. At night I could see lights from the mainland and Old Rhoades Key. The nighttime filled my van with moonlight.

The sun was strong, the temperature 85 degrees, and the breeze constant. Skinny-dipping and sunbathing were obligatory. I conjured up as many excuses as I could for hanging tight here. I couldn't have been happier if I had a million big ones in a Swiss bank and twenty-six pounds of red licorice. But after several days of this, I did put on my clothes and go back to work.

Almost all beekeepers use honey on serious burns, and many of them cited particular accidents they had had. But Dorian Wakefield told me the most dramatic story.

"When I first got into the bee business I was also working as a welder. I had an accident with the torch one day and burned an area on my left forearm here about three inches by five inches.

"The welding torch was at about 2,500 degrees and it just cauterized itself. I didn't even feel any pain for several hours. The hospital dressed the area and told me to come back in the morning.

"The next morning and thereafter I just put honey on that burn. A nice big scab formed, and it didn't flake off around the edges as most scabs do. When it was ready to come off, it just lifted right off and the skin underneath was pink and good.

"Look here, no scar."

And there wasn't a scar. There was no evidence that the arm had ever been burned.

In *Curative Properties of Honey and Bee Venom,* we find:

From his clinical observations, Dr. Krinitsky concluded that honey accelerates healing. He considers that honey, when applied to a wound, sharply increases the glutathione content in the wound secretion: glutathione plays a very important role in the oxidation-reduction processes of the body: it stimulates the growth and division of cells and in this way promotes the healing of wounds.

That night I woke up about midnight with an extraordinary pain in my left big toe. I don't have a very brave threshold of pain, and on my scale of one to ten it was maybe nine. Ten being the time I had bursitis in my hip. The pain came from the bone right to the last layer of skin, and it hurt to touch my toe. I thought at first it was gout, but there was no swelling. I couldn't sleep and daybreak was a long time coming. The night just ambled along like they sometimes do. In the morning I found a trigger point on the side of my toe, and it was inordinately sensitive. I knew what I had to do.

Back at Dorian Wakefield's I caught me a few bees and stung that trigger point five times.

The foot swelled considerably. I had some pain from the swelling. When the swelling went down after two days, I had no more pain and have not had any since. The trigger point is gone, and I believe the toe's going to be OK.

Several days before my visit with Mr. Ralph Wadlow, a hobbyist had told me that eating honey would cure bedwetting. Now I am really enthusiastic about my subject, but this claim went beyond credibility and bordered seriously on the absurd.

Mr. Wadlow is an apiary consultant to the Colombian government and has been a professional beekeeper most of his adult life. He told me the same thing. Has he perhaps taken one sting too many? Not so. Try this on for size.

From Ioyrish's *Bees and People:*

A teaspoon of honey before bed is recommended for babies cutting teeth. It reduces the amount of phosphorus in the blood and so eases the pain.

A similar dose of honey prevents bed-wetting, as it causes dehydration and reduces the amount of calcium in the blood.

Mr. Wadlow also told me that when he was a young man in the bee business he had an elderly neighbor who had cancer of the lip. He would come over and get honey from time to time to apply to his lip. He said it was the only thing that would give him relief from the pain.

Ira Powers and I were sitting in the shade of a steel building talking bees and arthritis. He had just come back from moving a mess of bees from an orange grove. There were half a dozen veiled young men about. I noticed presently that there were more and more bees in our immediate vicinity. I've got a wild bunch of black/gray (or is it gray/black?) wiry hair. Pretty soon I had a considerable number of bees in my "bonnet."

"Don't slap at them, Fred. Hold still. I'll get them out."

And Ira did get them out. All but two, and they got me good. One above the right ear and the other about where my forehead ends (or maybe commences—whatever).

Mr. Powers apologized. I waved the apology aside with: "Not to worry, it goes with the territory, but I believe I'll git on down the road." Foremost in my mind was Dr. Bodog Beck's claim that a sufficient quantity of alcohol (or in another manner of speaking, a good belt of booze) is an excellent way to neutralize the effects of bee venom.

By the time I was able to get a decent distance from the Powers's apiaries, the old head was tingling and getting plenty tight.

Fortunately, I had a modicum of Scotch in my pantry for just such emergencies, and I downed my medicine with dispatch. In fifteen minutes all sting sensations had ceased. It didn't pass the FDA's double- and triple-blind control test, but it sure suited me.

As pleasant as the remedy was, I determined to hide my bush under a straw hat when next the bees and I commingled.

"Do you sell cappings?" I asked Harold Curtis.

"I used to sell cappings to health food stores. People who ate them claimed it helped their sinus."

"Is that right? I know people use it for allergies and asthma, but I didn't know about sinus."

"Cappings for sinus and hayfever, really helps. And bought in the local area I know it helps you."

In the October 15, 1969, *Florida Farmers Bulletin:*

An Oklahoma allergist told a meeting of 150 beekeepers that raw honey is an effective treatment for 90 per cent of all allergies. Dr. William G. Peterson, an allergist from Ada, said he now has 22,000 patients across the nation who are using raw honey—along with more customary medication—to relieve allergic symptoms.

"It must be raw honey, because raw honey contains all the pollen, dust and molds that cause 90 per cent of all allergies," he told a meeting of the Oklahoma Beekeepers Association.

"What happens is that the patient builds up an immunity to the pollen, dust or mold that is causing his trouble in the first place."

"The raw honey must not be strained, not even through a cloth," he added. "I know the customer wants good, clear, strained, filtered honey, and that's fine, but for health reasons, raw honey is what we need."

Dr. Peterson said he and the 20 doctors at his clinic at Ada normally prescribe a daily teaspoon of raw honey. The honey treatment continues even after the allergy is under control.

It was late Sunday afternoon in La Belle and Harold had promised to take his son waterskiing so he had to scoot off. He invited me to come back in the morning. I spent the night alongside a canal running from the Gulf of Mexico through Lake Okeechobee to the Atlantic. I enjoyed a glass of beer and a sandwich and watched some fine waterskiing.

The next day in the Curtis's shop the employees and I had a little session.

"It's great for water on the knee too. I know an old guy who does it for water on the knee. Puts a sting right on the knee and it gets rid of the water. Takes about a day and it's back to normal."

It was dinnertime. Mr. A.C. Colson and his family reluctantly accepted the fact that I had just eaten and insisted I sit with them while they enjoyed their meal. Mr. Colson is a minister and a beekeeper. His voice has the dialect and timbre of Billy Graham's.

"I worked in a lumberyard for about fifteen years—thirteen years of that I spent in the office. They had a large air conditioner and they kept all of the office cold. In the summertime it's hot outside, eighty or ninety degrees, and when you go inside they got it cooled down to sixty—quite a contrast.

"And my job was in and out all the time. I developed arthritis. It was in my hands, in my fingers. I got to the point I couldn't even hold a pencil to write a ticket, figure an estimate. Finally, I had to quit.

"I was around home not knowing what to do with myself, not knowing what to do with the arthritis. I went down to the barbershop while I was waiting, not knowing what to do, and there are three or four men talking about problems. I said, 'What'd you do about arthritis?'

"Everything was quiet as it could be for a few moments. The barber stopped and bumped his comb on his scissors a time or two and said, 'Eat plenty of raw honey.' I said, 'Man, you got to be kidding.' He said, 'Try it.'

"Of course, then I didn't know anything about bees, and so I started out looking. Finally found an old beekeeper over here and bought a gallon of honey. I took it home and the whole family used it. It took us a month or so to eat it. I couldn't feel it had done any good. But I decided I'd give it a good try anyway, so I went back and got us another gallon. By the time that second gallon of honey was gone, I could tell my arthritis was better. So I said maybe there is something to it. I went back and bought two gallons. By the time we had used up the two gallons of honey, I almost didn't know I had had the arthritis."

"How old were you then, Mr. Colson?"

"I was about forty-eight or forty-nine. Since it worked I just sat down and wrote me an order to the A.I. Root Company for a colony of bees.

"I stood them up in my backyard, and people passing by would say, 'Hey, you can get a swarm of bees over there,' 'Hey, would you like to get these bees?' First thing you know I had sixty colonies of bees in my backyard."

Mrs. Colson also has some strong feelings about honey.

"Several years ago, I don't know how many ago, I had arthritis so bad in my shoulders and arms I couldn't hang up my clothes."

"And honey did it?"

"Honey and vinegar and water. An old colored lady said, 'If you'll take it just like I tell you to take it, it'll stop it.' Well, I'd been hurting, and medicine hadn't done no good. I couldn't go out and put my laundry on the line without hanging up a few pieces and then getting my arm down where the circulation would get to it.

"She told me just take equal parts of vinegar and honey in water. I'd take it every day just like that and within three weeks I could use my arms. It seems impossible. I didn't believe it, but I'd got to the point where I would have tried almost anything."

"Even bee stings?"

"Yessir, bad as I'm scared by them."

Mr. Colson was exactly right when he said, "When God made the bee he made a wonderful creature, and beekeeping is one of the most fascinating things I ever got into."

Here's a journal note you may find interesting:

March 21, 1977

Had a chat with a woman (twenty-five to twenty-eight) who worked for a local beekeeper—said bee stings cured her tennis elbow in just a month—also that she had freaked out too much on acid, her subconscious had developed and her conscious was suffering. She felt this was common among acid takers. She also felt strongly that honey was rebuilding her conscious—and making her horny. It was noontime and she invited me to share chilled fresh orange and grapefruit sections covered with honey. Nice!

Before leaving Florida I want to tell you a story I heard from one of Al Purkis's honey customers—a man from Maine.

"I knew this old farmer who had arthritis in his hands something fierce. Every once in a while when he couldn't function anymore he'd go out to the electric fence, grab onto it with both hands, and hold on for a few seconds. Then he'd let go and flex his fingers a few times and go about his business. Saw him do it a couple of times."

I believe I'd rather take a few stings!

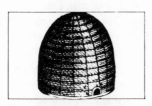

ELEVEN

MANY OF THE state and provincial campgrounds are singularly attractive, but some of them border on the disgraceful. I've been ripped off more times by California state parks than I care to recount. No electricity, no hot water, no flush toilets—and all this "nothing" for four dollars a night for one person.

You will therefore understand my joy at finding Clarke State Park near Stonewall, Mississippi. A level asphalt pad with water and electricity bordering a sandy beach and a natural lake. Lots of space between the pads and lots of tall pines. Hot showers in a heated room. It is class all the way, and I couldn't find a fee schedule or a place to pay. Shame on you, California.

This morning, rather than my usual quick, low-cost McMuffin at McDonalds, I opted for bacon, eggs, and grits at a truck stop in Scooba, Mississippi.

I had a good visit with the perky waitress, commenting on how beautiful I found this part of Mississippi. She told me the local government leaves you alone to do as you please in Scooba. That was a refreshing concept—one I thought was extinct. I remembered Vermont being like that in the early sixties. She also said it got so hot in the summer that the earth split open. So I stopped my questions about land prices. When I left I told her she was the prettiest grandmother I ever met. She was. I think I may have put some new colors in her paintbox that day.

Have you noticed that we are passing more and more laws to restrict the rights of the law abiding and more and more laws to protect the rights of the criminals?

Mayhew, Mississippi, is not easy to find. Nevertheless, Mr. P.A. Yelverton and a formidable number of bees know where Mayhew is. His apiary employs forty people year-round and seventy during the bloom. Coming from the east on 82 you may find a small sign if you have quick eyes. There's no sign coming from the west (which I was).

Nevertheless, take a dirt road over the tracks and you're into Mayhew, which is essentially the Stover Apiaries. It's the biggest operation I've seen. They don't sell honey. They sell bees and lots of them.

"I have arthritis," Mr. Yelverton said, "but I have the swelling arthritis, and I think bee stings don't help it. I think there are some kinds of arthritis that are helped by the use of bee stings. You get temporary relief, but at the same time relief is relief.

"I think that Certo, apple-cider vinegar, and honey benefits my swelling arthritis."

"You do?"

"Yes, I do. I take it when I need it."

"How do you take it? Do you take it in equal portions?"

"Right. Mix them together and take a tablespoon every morning and a tablespoon every evening till you begin to get relief, and then shut it off. People I talk to, eight out of ten benefit."

"How about any other use for bee products, Mr. Yelverton?"

"You can heal a sore quicker with honey or with royal jelly than with your so-called miracle drugs."

"Ever know a beekeeper to die of cancer?"

"Not that I know of. I tell you what I can tell you. People that are heavy eaters of honey generally live five to fifteen years longer than most people and they're sexually reproductive longer."

"Is this some documented stuff you've read that I could get my hands on?"

"Not the sexual bit, but I've just noticed it in beekeepers as a whole. We just loaded a man up this morning who is seventy-three, driving his truck, going, doing everything. He's overweight. That's all that's wrong with him."

"He's a beekeeper?"

"Full-time beekeeper. I know the Weavers over in Texas. They're both in their eighties and their mother lived to be 102 or 103 and she was a beekeeper from eight or nine or ten years old."

"I've met more than several in their eighties, and they seemed to be going strong," I said.

"Honey's a wonderful commodity. When you have problems going to sleep at night, if you take a spoonful of honey and say your prayers, you'll probably be asleep real quick.

"I'll soon be sixty-three and I do full-time work. In fact, in the rush season we quit about eight or nine o'clock at night and I'm up at five every morning, so I figure something has got to help you. Sure do."

"I won't hold you up any longer. Sure do appreciate your talking with me."

"Enjoyed it. Thank you and come back."

You can skip the next several pages if you've a mind to because there's not much going on, beewise.

I bedded down for the night on a U.S. Army Corp fishing boat ramp between Wax and Snap, Kentucky. I lay there looking at the stars and reflecting on this day's work. Mr. P.A. Yelverton had a sign on his office wall: "There's Nothing Me and the Lord Can't Handle Today."

Sometimes I believe in God. Sometimes I don't. But even when I don't, I strongly believe in the power of prayer to make things happen. Not all things—like making it rain or stopping a flood—but things like curing a cancer, leading a loved one to safety, or salvaging a derelict. In other words, people miracles.

Even those times when I believe in God, I cannot believe that if God permits war, famine, and pestilence he would at the same time concern himself with personal miracles that do an infinitesimal bit of good in the total scheme of things.

I think I know the answer. Science has long known that the subconscious section of the brain is much larger, more complex, and more potent than the conscious part. We know there is mental telepathy occurring between some minds frequently and most minds sporadically. These communications have to be between subconscious minds.

Generally prayers are not answered until the person praying is at the very depth of despair and his state of mind is, "God, I've done all I can do, I can do no more. I put myself in your hands."

A chemical/electrical action takes place whereby the conscious surrenders to the subconscious, which takes control at that point. The subconscious can then wield a great force over the person praying if he is praying for himself or can communicate directly with the subconscious mind of another person or group of people and get them to act or react.

This power to unleash the force of the subconscious is not necessarily restricted to the doing of good deeds. Voodoo may have discovered its own key, and this may account for the misery successfully visited upon its victims.

Now that I got that off my mind, I turned off the stars and went to sleep.

A few days later I was twenty miles south of Washington, D.C. It was 6 A.M. and I was on my way to the great repository of knowledge—the Library of Congress. Surely here would be an abundance of material on bee venom and honey.

I had started early in order to beat the traffic, but thousands of others clearly had the same idea and so the superhighways were choked.

I was most agreeably surprised by the spring beauty of the Potomac and the capital buildings. I gawked once too often, made a wrong turn within a block of the library, and next thing I knew was back on the Virginia side of the Potomac, heading south.

It took me a half hour to recoup my position. I planned on being at the library at least several days and determined I was not going to fight the same herd every morning. I found an all-night liquor store one block from the library and parked in front of it, under a street lamp. I figured the police would watch the place like hawks. Except for the sirens, I slept well.

There was a book by the Englishwoman, Julia Owens, titled *Doctors Without Shame,* describing some of her experiences with the medical profession and its attitude toward bee venom therapy. She recounts numerous cases in which doctors or their family members came to her for relief or cure by bee venom therapy and their subsequent refusal to publicly acknowledge that they had benefited from the therapy. It is an angry book and justifiably so, if accurate.

I checked the *Materia Medica* from 1970 to the present. This is an annual cumulative index of the scientific papers printed worldwide. Once, perhaps twice, each year, there was a listing of an American publication on the therapeutic uses of a bee product. On the other hand, there were dozens of papers each year published in foreign countries. I was not surprised, just disappointed.

On May 19, 1974, there appeared in the *Washington Post* a comprehensive account by Patrick Frazier titled "Arthritis and Bees." It is a splendid article and should be the first one you seek out. Following are some of the highlights I've extracted:

In 1962, a retired vice president of General Electric, Glenn B. Warren, established with his wife and sons a foundation for arthritis research in areas not being funded by other organizations. . . .

He ran a computer search of the literature on bee venom and soon met Benton, Broadman, Mraz and several others experienced with it. Warren decided that the treatment had potential, even though he knew it was too late for bee venom to help his own condition substantially.

He was not universally impressed, however, by how the treatments were handled. Some said there were trigger points that had to be stung or injected; others claimed that the venom's action is systemic and can be effectively injected anywhere. Some said BV therapy was sufficient; others said it had to be supplemented.

Unfamiliar with the professional and governmental complexities involved, Warren has spent the last six years trying to overcome the tinge of quackery that bee venom acquired among medical people, the disinterest of drug companies committed to producing synthetic steroids and the rigorous FDA protocol for new drugs. . . .

Maj. Vick has been able to confirm the beneficial action of bee venom in a second series of tests on 20 new dogs, 10 of which are control animals. The tests so far, lasting more than 30 days, have reaffirmed the increased cortisone output, and the arthritic dogs' mobility has increased an average of 50 per cent, their cage activity matching that of the nonarthritic animals.

Most enthusiastic about the tests, Warren remarks, "In front of a great many doctors who should know, I made the statement that, so far as I know there is no other instrumentality in the medical profession that has the ability to stimulate and maintain a high level of cortisone over a long period of time. And I've never been refuted or contradicted." Dr. Decker concurs, saying that this is "so unique as almost to be unbelievable. I'm unaware of any other compound that sustains cortisone at the level Vick has shown in his tests."

Bee venom's biggest challenge came after Warren talked Dr. Gerald Weissmann, professor of medicine at New York University's School of Medicine and one of the most respected researchers in rheumatology, into testing Mraz' bee venom on the adjuvant arthritic rat model, the standard model by which new treatments are tested. Everyone close to the bee venom work held their breaths at this point and Dr. Weissmann admits, "I thought it wouldn't work, frankly."

But after the first series of tests, an enthusiastic letter from him to Warren dispelled the doubts. Dr. Weissmann's tests ultimately showed that whole bee venom, more than its individual constituents, did suppress adjuvant arthritis when the rats were injected twice daily from the day the arthritis was induced.

Unlike many other drugs, bee venom prevented the arthritis from appearing after the injections were stopped, and it caused no adverse side effects. Apparently unaware of Dr. Weissmann's work British researchers also reported recently in Nature Magazine that they had discovered an anti-inflammatory element in bee venom they named Peptide 401. In working with the adjuvant arthritic rat, they too observed that arthritis did not develop after injections were stopped.

Offsetting the optimism of Dr. Weissmann's findings was the fact that when the same dose was given 17 days after the arthritis was established at a moderately severe stage, it did not turn back the disease. How then to account for the many dramatic and lasting benefits claimed by bee venom practitioners remains to be settled in human cases.

Nevertheless, Warren asserts, "I am convinced that for arthritis of relatively recent origin—five to 10 years or less—we can demonstrate a simple, inexpensive and largely effective treatment." Looking at Vick's and Dr. Weissmann's work, confirming bee venom's action through the pituitary gland to the adrenals, Warren says, "Now to me, as an amateur, this meant we might have, with bee venom treatment, eliminated one of the major problems associated with either ACTH or cortisone treatment of arthritis."

He refers to the tendency, with prolonged use of artificial steroids, toward atrophy of the body's own adrenal and pituitary glands. With bee venom, "We think we are working through the pituitary and the adrenal and not atrophying either of those. Now that would be all right, possibly, if we act in such a way that we don't atrophy something ahead of the pituitary—hypothalamus or something of that kind. But there has never been any evidence that old beekeepers—and there are millions of them in the world who've had a lot of bee stings—suffer the kinds of diseases that characterize people who have had an excess of either ACTH or cortisone treatment artificially."

Armed with the new scientifically acceptable studies and hoping to get help with successive and more expensive FDA requirements, Warren gathered together Vick, Dr. Weissmann, Mraz and Dr. Decker in February, 1973, to meet with representatives of Abbott Chemical Co., Dr. Charles Sisk from the Arthritis Foundation and the new deputy director of NIAMDD, Dr. Lamont-Havers.

Warren got little response from the Abbott men, but Drs. Sisk and Lamont-Havers pledged help in finding sponsors for clinical trials and offered their institutions' professional expertise in pursuing a program. Considering the controversy of 10 years previous, this represented quite a turnabout for bee venom. Dr. Sisk remarked, "Vick's study particularly is outstanding work on those dogs and I think it demands further trials."

According to Dr. Sisk, the Arthritis Foundation has agreed to set aside funds contributed which are specifically designated for bee venom research.

Dr. Weissmann thinks that getting a definitive answer to bee venom's potential requires determining the various actions its constituents have on an organism. And each constituent to be tested on a patient would have to pass the entire FDA basic training. Proper research, in his estimation, would entail five good clinical labs spending more than $100,000 each for two years, with patients tested toward the end of these studies.

Dr. Decker is cautious about bee venom's potential, but thinks it warrants investigating, even if it promises to be just another treatment. "It's my view," he explains, "that we, at this juncture, do need carefully designed studies of rheumatoid arthritis treated with bee venom. I would think that a pilot project involving 30 patients for maybe three or four months would be a very important factor in changing the opinions of lots of people, if he (Warren) got a solidly positive result out of such a study."

Dr. Weissmann observed that in the adjuvant rats' complicated biological response to bee venom, there appeared the possibility that its arthritis suppression may act in another, undetermined fashion aside from the pituitary-adrenal stimulation. It's conceivable then that this other mode of action, once pinned down, may clarify what is attracting the inflammation in the first place, and thereby help in discovering the disease's cause. "It looks awfully promising," Dr. Weissmann says, "but it's in a rudimentary stage."

Shipman and others found that 80 per cent or more of mice injected with bee venom survived when exposed to a lethal dose of radiation 24 hours afterward. Other compounds to be effective as radiation protectors have to be administered just prior to irradiation. Here, too, bee venom is operating in an unknown manner, different from all other compounds, and could provide clues to how the body protects itself.

Hopes are that it may aid in radiation treatment for cancer, if it doesn't protect cancerous cells as well as healthy ones. Lack of funds and facilities halted Shipman's and a coworker's experiments that hinted bee venom may have a positive place in leukemia research.

In work on isolated dog and monkey hearts, Maj. Vick and Shipman discovered a new BV constituent they named cardiopep, which has a pronounced stimulating and stabilizing effect, lasting much longer than other known drugs. This may offer hope to those who suffer from congestive heart failure.

"You know that when you get this damnable disease, your life span is probably about five years, even with the best drugs," according to Vick. "If cardiopep works as well as it appears to work and is as non-toxic now as Bill thinks it is, then we've got something that may double or even triple that life span."

"We now have it completely purified and isolated and we've tested it," Vick says.

One remarkable experiment concerns a chimpanzee that was in the throes of death from a lethal shock. Respiration had ceased and the heart was undergoing a faint fibrillation when Vick injected cardiopep. The chimp's heart and pulse rate began to stabilize, and after another injection two hours later, the chimpanzee returned to normal and stayed healthy.

Bee venom fans are not surprised by these side effects. They claim to have observed many improvements in maladies other than arthritis.

Dr. Terc, for instance, noticed a hundred years ago that two of his patients' heart irregularities ceased after bee sting treatment. Ironically, it's been claims like these that convinced most scientists that bee venom was one of those untrustworthy folk panaceas. But scientific preliminaries have so far confirmed much of what honeybee advocates maintained all along. Warren and Mraz have succeeded in focusing attention on an exciting "new drug," but getting things farther requires more people who will listen and help.

In the foyer of the Library of Congress is a Gutenberg Bible. About sixty feet away is a glass case with a copy of the *New Yorker* magazine showing a cartoon involving the library.

In 1967 I ran a real estate ad in the *New York Times*'s classified section. The *New Yorker* put some new toys in my playpen by reprinting the ad five years later and adding its own editorial comment:

> CHESTER—Abandoned gold mine on 50 acres with 2500′ frontage on Williams River, a glittering, gold flecked piece of business that pirouettes spiritedly with a gravel road named Smokeshire. A whimsical thing at $12,000. Fred Malone, Chester, Vt. 602/875–2381 or 362–2098 after vespers.—*Adv. in the Times.*
>
> After vespers all the whimsey's gone out of us.

I hope you will pardon me if my immodesty is a bit unseemly. But if the Library of Congress can brag about being cartooned in the *New Yorker,* I expect I can brag about some advertising copy it chose to ennoble.

That's the second good thing.

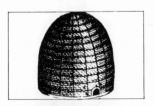

TWELVE

We were sitting on the deck facing the Hudson River. Everything seemed to be OK. Although Dr. Vogel was not "on call" this Sunday, he had left word with his clinic to let certain calls come through. Patients called rather frequently, and the doctor would pop up and talk a bit. I built a chalet for him in 1965 on a piece of Vermont land that I called "Finbar's Forest." That's how we became friends.

There was just a tinge of apprehension in the air. His wife Franzi had had two new stainless-steel "hips" installed several months earlier. She responded beautifully at first, but a problem seemed to have developed just a few days before my arrival.

"You know, Fred, I've seen hundreds and hundreds of arthritics down through the years. And I've always had sympathy for them, as I think I've had for most of my patients. But I never truly realized the depth of despair some arthritics go through. I watched Franzi, in a matter of months, go from an effervescent, extroverted woman to a withdrawn, forlorn introvert, not interested in anything. I was helpless to do anything. I'll never feel the same again about a person with arthritis. I had to live close to it to see the psychic destruction it can do. But I don't think her present discomfort is anything serious. She probably has a low-grade virus infection which has settled in the new joint."

I thought to myself, "How very true that is." I've had close friends who suffered with arthritis and I think I've always had the feeling, "Well it's just a necessary cross some of us must bear."

Even after I started having aches in my knees I didn't really understand the psychic agony arthritics go through when they know they're not going to get better and will probably get worse.

But when I got that searing pain in my big toe in Florida, I spent a good part of the night wondering what the hell I was going to do with that toe if the bees didn't fix it. I learned that night something of the debilitating despair many arthritics have. And I knew then, most certainly, if doctors had this experience even they might try eating ground bees.

I have reviewed a great number of books on arthritis written by medical men. Of these, only Dr. Broadman mentions the mental trauma:

Crippling transformations may be the thing we see. What goes on in the sufferer's mind, God only knows. Inability to work and consequent economic hardship may cause a man embarrassment. And what can disease do to his pride? Worst of all, perhaps, is intense physical pain—of all things the hardest to describe.

April 18, 1977. Spent the day in Westport, Connecticut, with Dr. Mary Lovelace and a patient who had flown in that morning from Mississippi. I learned then that there is an FDA-approved widespread method of curing insect venom allergies by injecting the ground-up insect in serum form. This treatment runs over an eighteen-month period—and it is not very satisfactory. Sometimes it provides immunity and sometimes not. You may be immune one day, she said, and not the next.

The patient from Mississippi told me that just part of the venom from one wasp used to render him unconscious in less than five minutes. He had been through the eighteen-month series, and it had not worked. Today, Dr. Lovelace had injected him with the full venom supply of six wasps. He probably would be immune in three to four days. Thereafter, he would be checked annually by Dr. Lovelace. He quite literally looked upon Dr. Lovelace as his savior because he had nearly lost his life several times by wasp stings.

Dr. Lovelace has successfully immunized over 400 people who were allergic to wasp stings. She applied to the FDA for approval of her technique, and they will not consider it until she has tested it on dogs. She said, "I've proved it on 400 people and they're all willing to come down and testify and you can test them for immunity." The FDA told her only the dog test would do.

She charges very modestly for this life-saving procedure. She has neither the money nor the time to comply with the FDA requirements. Maybe there's a Daddy Warbucks out there who would like to do something important with his money before he cashes in. But hurry. Dr. Lovelace, like you and even me, is not getting any younger.

Dr. Herman N. Sanders in New Hampshire had written a letter to Dr. Broadman which was reprinted in the latter's 1962 book. Was he alive and would he grant me an interview?

Yes, yes.

"Would you like a glass of beer or ginger ale or something like that?" Dr. Sanders asked.

"No, we're happy as clams. Matter of fact we just had a little lunch of honey and crackers."

Dr. Sanders is retired and now finds he needs twenty-five hours a day. He works one day a week covering the emergency room at the hospital. He also covers the county jail one or two days a week, he's on the Mosquito Control Board in New Hampshire and plays in a string quartet in Massachusetts.

"I don't think we have any cure for arthritis at the present time. All I know is that we have people who have acute arthritis—rheumatoid arthritis with the typical swollen joints, deformities, the weakness. There are specific ways of making the diagnosis of rheumatoid arthritis. Usually it's a bilateral affair. It's a systemic disease really. I've had several people like that who have been acutely ill, documented with rheumatoid tests, a blood test to determine sedimentation rate, which is a nonspecific test indicating the degree of involvement. The sedimentation rate is elevated with the acuteness of the illness. For all the people I've treated, I've usually followed their course with sedimentation tests because as they get better the sedimentation rate improves. It usually lags behind their improvement. Should they improve in, say, six weeks, their high sedimentation rate may go on for eight weeks, maybe ten weeks, before it completely gets down to normal again.

"But we've had several acute situations, for example people who were bedbound because the arthritis was so painful they couldn't walk. They couldn't do anything. We've put them through a course of treatments. One of these people was a veteran, in the Veterans Hospital. They had done everything with their aspirin and malaria pills, and they were just on the point of putting him through cortisone therapy. He happened to live in a small town beyond me and he said he had heard that I treated with the bee venom therapy and he'd like to try it.

"They discharged him and I saw him at home and treated him at home for about four to six weeks. About the third week he walked downstairs. We did tests on him, and by the end of six weeks he was back at work. I haven't seen him since, but he kept on working. I presume he still has arthritis of some sort.

"He was a veteran and I asked one of the leading doctors at the Peter Bent Brigham Hospital in Boston if he would come up here while I presented this to the hospital. At the same time, I invited the head medical man at the Veterans Hospital in Manchester [New Hampshire] to come out here also to see this case that I presented."

I asked him if they had accepted his invitation.

"Yes. They both shook their heads and said they didn't know, they didn't believe, they didn't know how it worked, but they didn't go along with it. They said they didn't believe it. They said, 'This is just one of those things that sometimes happens.'

"I have another lady that lives here, who met all the specifications for acute rheumatoid arthritis with bilateral involvement of several joints, elevated sedimentation rate, fever, fatigue. We put her through a course of treatment—this is over ten years ago—and she hasn't taken any medicines since that time. I happened to see her last week. She doesn't take aspirin; she's completely recovered. Now this was acute arthritis.

"They can say, and they probably will say, that a certain number of people with rheumatoid arthritis will make spontaneous recoveries. They may have an acute episode and they may not be bothered the rest of their life. But it's not the usual thing. It does happen, I'm sure.

"Over the fifteen or twenty years I treated patients—several hundred patients—I don't think there were over ten (and I can only think of five really) that didn't benefit from bee venom therapy. Now this is quite good when you think of over 400 or 500 people getting the therapy.

"The most dramatic bee venom results were in people who had acute bursitis—bursitis of the arm, where they were doing something and all of sudden they couldn't use the arm. If I could see such a person within twelve hours from the onset of the attack and I could give him one treatment, I would guarantee he would be able to raise the arm over his head. And this has happened every time as long as I catch them within the first twelve or twenty-four hours.

"I have over fifty people documented who had acute bursitis, and I cured every one of them. This was 100 percent of those who didn't drink any alcohol. I don't know any form of treatment—except possibly cortisone injections, which will almost do the same thing but are very painful for the first twenty-four hours."

I asked Dr. Sanders how successful he was if a patient delayed getting treatment beyond the twenty-four hours—say, for a week or more.

"I could get them all back. It would take more treatments, but I could get them all back."

"Within a week?"

"Yes, within a week. All the doctors would say, 'Why don't you write up all these things?' I'd say, 'I've been so busy I haven't had time to do any writing.' I practiced in the country, and I was just pooped at the end of the day. I wasn't in any position to write up my cases."

I mentioned to Dr. Sanders that his letter printed in Broadman's book speaks of bee venom ointment.

"Forapin has been put up in an ointment form. The last batch of ointment and serum I had come to this country from Germany was impounded by the government. I had to stop treating people."

"What was your experience with ointment? Did you get good results with that?"

"Yes. With an aching joint. It comes with a little file, like a nutmeg grater, to rupture the skin. So you roughen the skin a little bit and then you rub the ointment in. You get almost instant relief of a joint by putting Forapin on it."

I asked Dr. Sanders if he would be leery of using bee venom therapy nowadays with the high incidence of malpractice suits.

"I don't know. I've never worried about people with malpractice suits. I've always had a good rapport with people and I do the best I can with them. I really knocked myself out trying to take the best care of people, and how any of them could sue me . . . but I suppose there are people around who do things like that.

"But I have never had an ill effect from bee venom."

"Do you think the United States will ever come to know bee venom as an accepted means of therapy for arthritis?" I asked.

"Interesting thing. In England they're using it; in Russia they're using it; in some of the communist countries they're using it. In the United States, the big concerns have things going for them. They have cortisone going for them. They have aspirin going for them. They put out their malaria drugs, and they have other things. This is a manufacturing thing. If you all of a sudden come up with bee venom and it does a better job than any of these others and it's safe if you know how to use it—well, it has a place in therapy.

"But I couldn't get any of these people to go along with it. And they have the money and facilities that I didn't have for doing it. All I know is that I treated a lot of people and 75 to 80 percent are better. I don't know what other treatment would give as good results.

"They say you haven't done your double-blind or your triple-blind studies or whatever, and I accept that. The only problem is that these people get better. I don't promise them anything, and a large percentage of people get better. I was as skeptical of this as any doctor could be. I told Charlie Mraz he was crazy and not to bother me anymore. He badgered me until finally I tried it. If it hadn't worked, I would have been the first to quit. But it not only worked on the first patient, it worked on several after that. And I said, 'Lord sakes, maybe he's got something.' "

I asked Dr. Sanders if he had been in touch with the National Arthritis Foundation or any similar group.

"Yes I belonged to the American Rheumatic Diseases. I thought I could do some research in there and get some input. I went to many of the meetings. I talked to them and I could see them turning away from me, saying, 'There's another nut.' "

"Boy, that must have been frustrating."

"No, it wasn't frustrating. I accepted it. I expected it, so I wasn't frustrated. I expected it."

"Did you know Dr. Broadman?"

"Yes. He was trying to get a clinic set up in New York for treatment by bee venom. Some people had given him grants to do this. But he was thwarted every which way trying to get anything done. He was in his late years. He was very much upset because every way he turned he was thwarted."

"You must have gotten a great deal of satisfaction out of seeing the results of this work."

"I did. I still have people who call back to ask if I'm still using bee venom. I tell them no, and they ask where they can get some. I was interested to learn from you that Forapin is still around."

"Yes, but in Germany."

"Their stuff is excellent."

My visit with Dr. Sanders had been useful and good. But I wondered again if I would live long enough to see American arthritics get help from the bees.

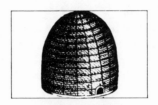

THIRTEEN

SALLIE WAS really intrigued with my stories about honey and health.

"Will honey cure hemorrhoids?"

"Beats me."

"Well, I'm going to try it on my trip down South."

A week or so later I got a card with the sole message: "Dear Fred: Honey relieves 'roids'! Love, Sallie."

I thought Sallie was putting me on. But a couple of days after I got the card I was up in Danby Four Corners, Vermont, looking for a beekeeper Sallie had told me about by the name of Roger Olson.

When I inquired about Roger's whereabouts, a tradesman directed me to an old-time beekeeper by the name of Roy Webster.

"He started using honey as an ointment."

"For what?"

"Hemorrhoids."

"Hemorrhoids?"

"Yep. Apparently its affinity for moisture must have absorbed the liquid. They shrank right down, and it was doing him more good, and he was living with it, than any other remedy he had ever used."

"Well, I'll be darned."

"I had a touch of hemorrhoids some years ago, and because of that, I used honey."

"Clear them up?"

"Cleared them up."

"Well, I'll be darned."

"His name was Hutchins. He's long since gone. Lived up Granville way. But I know he swore by it."

I don't have any hard evidence that honey will help hemorrhoids, but mixed half and half with Vaseline, it wouldn't hurt to try.

Jean Valetas received a French patent in 1968 on a medicament containing royal jelly, which is reputedly useful in the treatment of hemorrhoids.

And so it goes.

Here is a news clipping my friend Wilf Copping sent me that shook my socks:

In a recent letter to the *Resident and Staff Physician,* Dr. Gerald Glowacki, director of obstetrics and gynecology, Franklin Square Hospital, Baltimore, Md. comments that after vasectomies "About 25 percent of men develop antisperm antibodies. In these cases the body is required to lower its immunological resistance and thus becomes more susceptible to various maladies." Dr. Glowacki stated, "Recent reports show that post vasectomied males with sperm antibodies have developed significant arthritis and it is believed that susceptibility to such diseases as lymphoma, leukemias and Hodgkin's disease are all theoretical potentials of this sequence of immune events."

Now he tells me!

You will recall that the Victoria rheumatologist and I had determined that the pains in my knees may have been caused by arthritis in my back. That was Charlie Mraz's thinking, and he had said early on that was where the stinging had to be done. Now that I was back at Bob Richardson's in Vermont, he could help me do the stinging and I resolved to go at with purpose. Here are some excerpts from my journal:

April 20

> Stung myself seven times on the back. Put the ice on for a long time. Shook up seven bees in a jar, then Bob inverted it over the numbed area. The bees clung to the top of the jar and wouldn't land on my back. Bob thumped the jar and finally they were all walking around on my back but *not* stinging. Bob put some cardboard between them and the jar and pressed lightly. When they finally got around to stinging the numbness was gone and it hurt like hell! Just a little swelling. Slightly elevated heartbeat. Slept well.

I lay there on my stomach with those bees stinging the bejesus out of me and thought, "Why am I putting up with all this foolishness?" I remembered while breakfasting at McDonalds in Custer, Texas, reading the following newspaper account:

> Marion Pitchford, 56, of Charlotte, used his pocket knife to cut off part of his arm Wednesday night after it was caught and broken in a machine that sorts raw cotton fiber.
>
> Pitchford initially wanted to drive himself from the factory to the hospital. A co-worker offered to do the driving, but he did not have a license and had to stop after about a block because of his inability to drive.
>
> The men flagged down a cab but it had only gone about three miles before it was stopped by a flat tire. Pitchford was standing beside the cab on an access ramp to Interstate 77 when Sgt. M.D. Cooper of the Mecklenburg County Police Department spotted him.
>
> "When I pulled over and saw his arm, I told him to get in," Cooper said. "He said, 'I don't want to get blood all over your car.' I said 'Don't you worry about that. You just get in this car.' He's a tough old bird."
>
> He said he was in great pain when he cut his arm, but "I was most interested in getting out of that thing."

I guess that's it. I am interested in getting out of arthritis.

April 21

Used ethyl chloride, but the freezing effect only lasts seconds and so it did no good. Hurt again, a lot. Seven stings—no elevation of heartbeat. Slight swelling. Good sleep. No discernible improvement in knees. Slight ache around swollen area.

April 22

Stung myself ten times in a spot on my back that seemed to have two pressure (trigger) points. Unlike the other two stingings, this developed a solid red circle. Well, let's hope for the best.

April 23

Used the block of ice—left it on until I couldn't feel it anymore. First five stings I couldn't feel at all, next five I did feel, but not terrible severe.

April 27

Couldn't get any bees until today because of the rain. Stung my back sixteen times—used the ice in two applications—hardly felt a thing.

Between April 19 and May 12 "Doctor" Bob stung my back 211 times. My knees were still not right, and I was pretty down in the mouth.

May 15

Had pains from left foot up to my knee—outer edge. First time I've had pains between those two points. Maybe the pain in the knee originates in the foot. Found three trigger points and stung second, third, and fourth toes. Pain in the knee disappeared.

May 16

Right knee bothered today and then the left. Also both feet. Found trigger points in both feet and stung right foot four times and left three times. Pain went away in both knees. Wouldn't that be something if it's my feet that are causing the problem and I can keep finding the trigger points to sting?

I had a very pleasant Sunday afternoon visit with my friends Mort and Jean Julius. With some reluctance I had embarked on my wondrous bee venom and honey tales. I say with reluctance because Jean is head nurse at the Green Mountain Health Clinic and I had become rather sensitive to the frosty reception the medical fraternity had given me from time to time when recounting my "spooky" stories.

Not so with Jean. She has the open mind of all truly intelligent people. Furthermore, she added to my honey lore by telling me that the clinic uses honey to treat troublesome cases of bedsores, with great success.

The assumption is that a person who survives all the regimens, academics, and toil required to become a doctor has intelligence at least somewhat above the norm. The encyclopedia doesn't say so, but I choose to think that part of the baggage of intelligence is a finely honed curiosity and open-mindedness. I feel certain that people begin their medical studies with these worthies. What a shame, both for us and for them, that somewhere along the line so many lose these precious qualities.

Here is an appropriate (and maybe helpful) quotation from Dr. Joe D. Nichols's book, *Please, Doctor, Do Something!*:

It is not uncommon for a medical man to push back the waves of ignorance as a result of a personal experience. Dr. James Greenwood, Jr., clinical professor of neurosurgery at Baylor University's College of Medicine in Houston, told a scientific symposium how his golf game was being destroyed by a back disc problem that also brought him severe lumbosacral pain. But he had read somewhere that vitamin C would help his condition, and he started taking large doses of the vitamin. The pain disappeared. He resumed his golf game. Then, as an experiment, he stopped taking vitamin C. The back pain returned. Next, he resumed vitamin C therapy. The pain again vanished. . . .

Dr. Greenwood told the symposium of scientists in 1964, "With our increasing knowledge, the understanding of the intricacies of the chemistry of the body becomes more hopeless. This does not mean that present knowledge should not be used to its greatest extent, but it does indicate that one should not be forced to wait for complete scientific knowledge before using methods of treatment which are not harmful and which show hope of success."

My lady Jeannie, back in British Columbia, had become aware of the beneficial effect of honey on the complexion. She found the stickiness hard to handle, so she mixes honey and Vaseline in equal portions and uses this for a nightly facial and for chapped hands and lips.

One day, her son, Kier, came home with a painful sunburn on his back. She applied the Vaseline-honey concoction, and the stinging disappeared almost immediately.

Ace Waite, a Vermonter, told me he had come down with arthritis in his knees so badly that he couldn't even cross a trout stream. That was in August 1960.

His older sister told him to eat honey and lots of it. He did. He went hunting in November and he was well enough to drag a buck half a mile out of the woods.

He said that once he gave up honey for a while because he wanted to lose weight. The arthritis came right back on him. He threw calories to the wind, got back into honey, and the arthritis cleared up.

My daughter Judi is a secretary at the Vermont Country Store, which is only a short shoot from Bob Richardson's house. Almost every day I wheeled my van to Weston, and we would lunch in my "dining room."

The day her boss, Lyman Orton, returned from his holidays, she was skittish to beat all. She asked me if I had anything to help her relax. I told her I could give her a Valium, but why not "pop a pollen tablet down the old pipe and see what kind of tunes the organs play?"

She did and that night at dinner she told me it really relaxed her. Now she and spouse Steve take them every day. She says he's positively grouchy until he gets his pollen pill.

The following quote is from *Apitherapy Today:*

Consequently, it can be asserted directly that the effect of pollen is not universal, but it must be noted that it exerts a favourable influence upon the digestive and intestinal functions, restores the appetites, fights the most rebellious states of weakness, refractory to any other treatment, that it can contribute to the cure of neuroses and psychical depression, neurasthenia, prostate diseases, diabetes and, moreover, it can restore the virility of those who have functionally lost it.

My son, Fred the Younger (I'm Fred the Elder) wheeled me over the mountain to lunch one day. We stopped in Londonderry, Vermont, at a health food store so I could replenish my pollen stores. The pert clerk showed me the only thing she had, a pollen/royal jelly combination. My son said, "You take that stuff, Pa, and you're not getting back in the car with *me.*"

Monica Porter and I were taking some sun in her backyard in Woodstock. I was telling her about the things I had done since we had visited with William Matson back in October—about how his claim that he had never known a beekeeper to die of cancer really spurred me on to do the book.

She complained of a sore throat she had had for days and couldn't shake. I sprang into action, for I had learned from dozens of beekeepers that sipping a concoction of honey, bourbon, and lemon juice would cure not only a sore throat but a lot of other stuff you didn't even know you had.

Now Monica thinks I have a fair share of smarts. Nevertheless, she was as skeptical as all get out because this treatment was too simple, and after all, "Isn't honey the same as sugar?"

She smoked her cigarette and sipped my potion and finally admitted after an hour or so that her throat was much better. It cleared up by evening.

I recommended the same thing to my friend Ian Grassick some months later, back in Victoria, and it worked. I even have him taking honey before bed every night, and he claims he's sleeping better than he has for a long time.

Do that for me now, won't you?

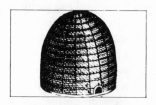

FOURTEEN

I ARRIVED at Dr. Joseph Saine's clinic at 7 A.M. My appointment was for nine, but since I did not speak French, I allowed myself plenty of time to get lost (and then found) in Montreal.

I sat in the hallway of his clinic and presently was introduced to his daughter, also a doctor, and a very warm, interested person. She served me a tall glass of apple cider they had made on their farm. She did not find it at all strange when I recounted the connection I had happened upon between my feet and my knees. I was happy to learn later that both she and her brother will be carrying on Dr. Saine's important work.

Dr. Saine's treatment for arthritis varies from those I had thus far studied in two essential areas. He not only injects bee venom serum intradermally, but for advanced cases he injects deep into the joints, muscles, and tissues. In addition, he uses a procedure called electrotherapy pioneered by d'Arsonval. This is an involved method of treatment that may employ short waves, infrared or ultraviolet rays, ultrasound, or ionization. Using diet, bee venom serum, and electrotherapy in various combinations, Dr. Saine feels that most arthritics can be significantly relieved if bone deformity has not set in.

Over the past seventeen years Dr. Saine has treated thousands of patients with apitherapy. Talking with Dr. Saine, reading his various addresses to the medical profession, and looking at the faces of the many patients who came into the clinic, I realized that he may very well be the world's most knowledgeable man about the treatment and cure of arthritis. I would not hesitate to put myself or my loved ones under his care. In fact, one of France's leading physicians sent his son to Dr. Saine, who cured him of arthritis.

I asked Dr. Saine if he knew the rheumatologist to whom I had been referred by the bee lab in Tucson. Yes, he did. Did he know how his research in bee venom was going?

Dr. Saine told me the research idea had been dropped. The research grants under which this rheumatologist functioned were made by drug companies. When they discovered that research was going to be done on bee venom, they threatened to stop the funding.

In an article in a scientific journal this same rheumatologist was quoted as saying: "With our current limited knowledge of this disease, we cannot completely ignore any lead—no matter how inconsequential it may seem at first."

No comment.

The pile of material Dr. Saine gave me on arthritis is too voluminous to repeat in total. Here are some excerpts that may be helpful to those of you who may want to try your own therapy.

From his September 12, 1976, lecture to the International Academy of Preventive Medicine, Kansas City:

I checked and found that if bee venom is injected along the cervical, dorsal and lumbar spine, I obtain better results than if it is injected in the buttocks or the arms. Second, I discovered the existence of a chain of painful spots along the vertebrae and around the articulations of the superior and inferior limbs. Following are certain characteristics of these painful spots:

1. They appear along the spine before appearing around the articulations of the limbs.

2. The patients usually are not aware of these painful spots, do not complain about them and, consequently, the doctor is not prompted to check them.

3. While the patient is being treated, the spots around the limbs disappear before those along the spine. It is nature's way to indicate where to inject and when to stop injecting.

4. In order to find the painful spots, the doctor has to use his middle finger or the reflex hammer.

5. The acuteness of the pain provoked by the hammer or the finger is in direct proportion with the acuteness of the disease or of the hypernervosity of the patient.

6. The appearance of all the painful spots is not simultaneous. If the arthritic patient presents a few painful spots only along the cervical column, the arthritis is just starting. On the contrary, if the painful spots are installed along the spine, it can be sure that mostly all the articulations of the patient are attacked and the arthritis is generalized.

7. There is no synchronism in the appearance of the hypersensitive spots, either in all the sections of the spine or at the right or left side of a section.

8. When all the sections of the spine and all the articulations of the limbs are attacked in the left and right sides and in the external and internal sides, then the arthritis is generalized and usually we are confronted with a rheumatoid arthritis with its present or potential deformations and with hypersedimentation and hyperpositiveness of the latex, RA and Rheumaton tests.

9. The appearance and disappearance of the hypersensitive spots indicate the beginning or the end of the crisis of the disease. Thus, we can consider that mother Nature has given us a sure method to establish diagnosis and prognosis of the arthritic diseases.

From Dr. Saine's address at the International Symposium on Apitherapy, Bucharest, in 1965:

Hence we forbid them to eat white sugar; [and] bread and pastry made of flour whitened with nitrogen peroxide and unbalanced in its composition by the extraction of the bran, minerals, B vitamins, part of its protein, and, especially, its wheat germ, a source of vitamin E.

We recommend general hygiene, including careful mastication and well balanced diet made up not only of proteins, lipids and glucides but also fruits and raw vegetables green and fresh. For white sugar we substitute honey; for tea and coffee, which, especially when taken during the evening, interfere with sleep and produce a state of vaso constriction, we substitute herb teas and often linden-blosson tea with honey. Note that ordinary tea is constipating.

From his lecture at the University of Vermont:

My conviction is that we can prevent arthritis by a well balanced diet, by a strong physical activity or sports and by fighting against constipation and infections. . . .

But modern life with its cars, tractors, planes, machinery of all kinds, preventing man from walking and toiling; modern life with its canned food and white bread deprived of minerals and vitamins and made of flour sterilized with nitrogen peroxide; modern life with all those factors and others, induces to flatulence (gaseous), hemogliasis and constipation, lower temperature and capillary constriction and consequently to arthritis. . . .

Bee venom is a dissolvent of hyaluronic acid, a focal factor of arthritis. . . .

Because of its properties of stimulation on antehypophysis and the supra-renal glands, bee venom enhances the body defense, but, unlike cortisone, without dangerous side effects.

Bee venom is an anti-coagulant more active than hinudin and, thus, it diminishes the blood viscosity or hemogliasis and is useful even in certain heart conditions. . . .

With bee venom we did not only cure or relieve certain simple cases of rheumatism but also very chronic osteo-arthritis with deformities and even fibrous ankylosis. The osteofied ankylosed cases are the only cases we have not yet succeeded in resolving. . . .

What is the duration of the treatment? Some cases take two or three weeks; others 2–3 months; the cases with deformities and fibrous ankylosis, 1 year or even more. . . .

Can a cure be permanent? Yes. But we shouldn't forget that the same cause in the same circumstances can produce the same effect. That is to say, the relieved or cured patient does not acquire immunity. . . .

After 20 years of research on arthritis, neurological diseases and circulatory disorders, I have become more and more convinced that truth is simple and that man complicates life and even medicine. . . .

We physicians, whose task is to relieve suffering humanity, should understand that, to achieve our goal, the best rule to guide us should be to imitate nature: Nature is our mother, our master. . . .

I hope that very soon a great many North American universities will establish programs of biological research on bee venom as is being done in Europe and that the majority of our hospitals will use bee venom in arthritis, heart diseases, circulatory disorders, neurological and psychiatric dysfunctions. . . .

May I add that my collaborators all over the world as well as myself are confident that *truth will triumph and very soon.*

Hmmm. That address was given in 1962.

Mr. Paige was as great on the mound as Dr. Saine is in the world of medicine. I don't think the doctor would quarrel with the following.

SATCHEL PAIGE'S RULES FOR RIGHT LIVING

Avoid fried foods which angry up the blood.

If your stomach disputes you, lie down and pacify it with cooling thoughts.

Keep the juices flowing by jangling around gently as you move.

Go very lightly on the vices such as carrying on in society—the social ramble ain't restful.

Avoid running at all times.

Don't look back. Something might be gaining on you.

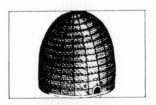

FIFTEEN

I was sitting in the office of Dr. G. Townshend, an entomologist with the University of Guelph in Ontario. Dr. Townshend certainly is one of the most knowledgeable people in the field of apiculture. And more important to me, he is a helpful man and rich in curiosity.

Dr. Townshend has done some outstanding work in the analysis of royal jelly. I asked him if he had any strong feelings about the therapeutic value of royal jelly.

"I don't think we have any evidence to show it is of any value yet. Really, there's no sound evidence; there are indications. I worked for pretty nearly ten years with a National Institute grant in this area.

"We had indications that one of the compounds in royal jelly had an effect on cancer cells, but it was passive—it didn't last long and, therefore, what we found afterward by labeling it with radioactive carbon was it was being broken down by the body of the animal into fat.

"We isolated this compound from royal jelly to show that it did have a passive effect on cancer cells. We found out why so when we blocked this, what we call beta—oxidation was taking place by substituting an oxygen for a carbon, and when we used it on cancer cells in the animal we found out it wasn't broken down but it did control the development of cancer cells. But this is the synthetic compound, similar to the one found in royal jelly.

"This, you see, is where a lot of these problems with these things come up. You have maybe a very slight effect, and this can lead to a discovery of something else that can be synthesized and that can be useful. This is where you get into many of the problems with natural compounds. They may have a slight effect but not enough to be useful, but it may lead to something else."

My mind flashed to March 5. I must write and tell young Meier in Paris, Texas, what use that Mexican royal jelly may be put to.

Wisconsin reminded me once again and repeatedly that I like cows. I mean I really like cows. I noticed when I was in real estate that when I sold a dairy farm it was always a sad time if the farmer had to sell off the herd. One of my "rose ladies," Clara Anderson, told me that farmers always individually name their cows. "They have their own personalities and they deserve their own names," she said. Clara had a 500-acre dairy farm that she pretty much ran herself. She ought to know. She knows a lot of other stuff too. She's a wise and wonderful woman.

My "rose ladies" were a bevy of ladies ranging from their midforties to late eighties. I would visit them on Christmas Eve and bring a rose instead of sending a Christmas card. Some I have known since I was eight. It took some time to see each of them for they were scattered about Vermont. But it was certainly worthwhile to me. A single rose, as I say, brings a lot of mileage.

At General Electric there was lower management, top management, and medium brown management. I mostly operated in medium brown. It used to crack me up the way the medium brown managers had loving family portraits all over their desks at the same time they were dicky dooing their secretaries. On my desk I installed a framed black-and-white photo of a host of holstein heifers hoofing down a hill. I smiled every time I looked at it.

Maybe that's why I didn't get that Denver promotion.

The Mayo Clinic has a very impressive aura about it—like being in a splendid, old cathedral. I was so nonplussed I gave several wrong/dumb answers to the receptionist. But I got to see the doctor I was seeking anyway.

He neither confirmed nor denied that the clinic had treated a woman with arthritis using bee venom serum. He just smiled.

His field was not rheumatology, but pediatrics and allergies. He has been using bee venom to treat bee sting allergies and had an investigational new drug license from the FDA to use bee venom. This license must be renewed every year. He showed me a copy of a report he must submit annually for license renewal. It was 8½ by 11 inches and fully 1 inch thick. Small wonder Dr. Lovelace cannot go through these machinations to get approval for her method.

The doctor paid me the compliment of asking me to send him any printed material I ran across that included blood and urine analyses being done on subjects treated with bee venom. This info would go into his 8½ by 11 report.

He gave me a photoprint of an article that appeared in *Industrial Medicine and Surgery,* titled, "Standardized Bee Venom Therapy of Arthritis," by Felix Steiger Waldt, M.D., Ph.D., Chief Physician, Third Medical Department, Municipal Hospital of Munich, Schwabing, Munich, Bavaria, Germany; H. Mathers, M.D., Assistant at Rheumatic Clinic, Medical University Polyclinic, Munich, Bavaria, Germany; and Frederic Damrau, M.D., Medical Research Consultant, New York City.

The report is based on use of a standardized isotonic bee venom solution (SBV) which is marketed in Germany and many other foreign countries under the name Forapin Standardized Bee Venom Solution.

Here is their summary:

A controlled clinical test of SBV in 50 cases of arthritis studied at two rheumatological clinics in Munich showed benefit in 84% of the treated cases as compared with 55% of the placebo controls. When the cases showing only slight improvement are deleted the rating for SBV is 66% as compared with 27% for the placebo. The improvement was manifest mainly by relief of pain but also increased joint mobility and disappearance of swelling and erythema.

The relatively good results obtained with the placebo provide an example of the fortuitous psychological factors often observed in the treatment of arthritis. Allowing for this discount, the favorable results obtained with SBV are nevertheless statistically significant.

It was observed that in patients under treatment with the cortico-tropic steroids, the doses may be reduced by the use of SBV, thereby lessening the hazard of their side effects.

A review of the literature on the apitherapy of arthritis, including the use of live bee stings and injectable preparations, shows that the consensus of medical opinion based on clinical investigations supports its value for palliative relief of the symptoms including pain, impaired mobility, swelling and redness.

That was the December 1966 issue.

Ed Honl, a Minnesota beekeeper, has been messing with bees more than fifty years. His whole family is involved in it. Strangely enough, one of his sons is allergic to dead bees. Live bees don't bother him a bit, but dead ones are bad news. Most people seem to hold the contrary view.

I asked Ed if he did anything with honey besides eat it.

"About thirty years ago Haydak told me about burns and honey. I never had real occasion to use it outside of the small stuff.

"Our oldest son—this goes back now at least twenty-five years ago—had a bicycle. He wanted me to make a hitch in the back to put a wagon on. In those days all you had for heating was one of those pump-up blow torches.

"Anyway, I heated up one piece of iron. It was a warm, muggy summer day. I laid it down and reached to pick up the other piece and instead picked up the one I had just heated.

"Believe it or not I heard that thing fry before I felt it. And just like that I thought of Haydak. So I ran in the house and stuck that hand in a pail of honey.

"Believe it or not I used that hand the next day. That's a fact. I'll never forget that."

"And there's no scar there?"

"No, I have no scars or nothing. I will never forget that. Never even blistered."

I spent several enjoyable evening hours with Ed Honl talking about bee people I had met in the last several months. He knew many of them. We had some coffee and cookies.

Winthrop, Minnesota, is a town of about 2,000 people. I asked if the police would hassle me if I pulled off the road for some shuteye. Actually, I was angling for an invite to pull into his bee yard because I had heard three convicted murderers had escaped from the Stillwater Prison and were still at large.

"Nothing to worry about around here. Nobody will bother you. Nothing to worry about."

I looked over his Airstream trailer and he looked over my van. He said I must be a shipwright. He expressed joyous approval of my bumper sticker, "Honey Lovers Stick Together," and once again I was sorry to leave a beeman.

It was late when I finally spotted a good berth in an alfalfa field some place between Winthrop and Minneapolis. I had some Minnesota cheddar cheese and dark pumpernickel. I lusted for a smidgen of red wine to ease the comestibles down the old pipe. But I had fetched along a jar of bees from Vermont, and we know now that mixing venom and booze is taboo.

I stung each foot a couple of times and conjured thoughts that if I were ever discovered doing this in the middle of the night, in the middle of an alfalfa field with that luminous fluorescent glow in my bubble, I'd be put in the stocks for being a warlock for sure.

I unrolled my four inches of foam, climbed under my eiderdown quilt and into the "Biological Bases of the Therapeutic Use of Bee Venom," by Professor N.M. Artemov, Chairman, Department of Physiology, Faculty of Medicine, National University of Gorki, USSR. This is a thought-provoking work. Its essence is that bee venom stimulates a mammal's immunological system to fight disease successfully.

It is forty pages long, which I will spare you because we're both tired. But here is some stuff I've extracted. Remember these are highlights only and taken out of context:

It is regrettable that the therapeutic use of bee-venom in most cases has been empirical. This results in many errors and contradictions and gives rise to all kinds of foolish opinions. It stands to reason that the most important task is to elaborate a biological theory which deals with the physiological action of bee-venom on the organism and it should completely explain the complicated symptoms of irritation, the cause of the variations in the threshold of reactivity, as well as the prophylactic and therapeutic characteristics of bee-venom. This task appears to us to actually be more important than the collection of clinical and experimental achievements; it should be done before trying to establish a bond between these achievements and their synthesis, as well as their theoretical explanation. . . .

This biologically active protein possesses most of the pharmacological qualities of venom. It has been named "Mellitin" and one considers it the most active substance of bee-venom. . . .

Its most remarkable quality is its capacity to block the transmission of nerve impulses from one cell to another in the ganglions of the nervous vegetative system, i.e., to block the transmission of nervous impulses (gangliolytical action).

Mellitin, also, acts on blood circulation in the organism. Upon its introduction into the circulatory system, one observes a decrease in the arterial pressure due to a dilation of the capillary vessels. Furthermore, it possesses an irritating action and provokes an inflammatory reaction upon its introduction into the skin or on the surface of mucous membranes. We may suppose that the therapeutic action of venom depends on this protein. . . .

Bee-venom has evolved to the point of acting on the most important and most vulnerable systems—the nervous system, the blood system, etc. On the other hand, this has forced the mammalian organism to develop reactions, which permit it to fight against the toxic effects of venom. . . .

During the evolution-process, bee-venom has become a natural stimulant and specifically capable of mobilizing the defense-mechanism which has been developed during the evolutionary fight of the organism against the bee. In reality, the dominating symptoms in envenomation are the expression of the activity of these defense-forces.

Contrary to certain chemical agents, which the mammalian organism has not encountered in the course of its evolution, bee-venom is a specific, powerful stimulant, which, in small quantities provokes a very complex "standard defense reaction," which can, otherwise, only be provoked by an action as powerful as a serious traumatism, a burn, or by bacterial toxins. . . . We should always remember the double action of bee-venom: it attacks the vital systems of the organism and in turn mobilizes the organism's defense forces. . . .

This indicates strong stimulation of the secretory activity of cortico-adrenals. Even relatively weak doses of venom (3 stings) produce a very considerable effect. . . .

We were able to affirm that bee-venom is a powerful stimulant of the adrenal system and that this fact plays a great role in the syndrome of envenomation by bee-venom. . . .

Among the people who systematically receive bee-venom, the phenomenon of cross-immunity resistance to other toxic agents is very interesting to study. The resistance of beekeepers to certain sicknesses (confirmed through statistical data) can probably be explained by this increase in cross-immunity. It is interesting in the same chain of reasoning to note the following verifications of many statements by clinical physicians. At the start of the treatment, the sick person, who suffers from arthritis or other sicknesses, reacts slightly to bee-venom. During the treatment, the reactivity of the sick person changes and amelioration corresponds, habitually, to an increase in sensitivity to the venom. . . .

Thus, in the treatment of polyarthritis, one recommends strong dosages of venom, whereas, in bronchial asthma one has to use smaller doses of venom. . . .

The following sicknesses are pointed out as suitable for bee sting treatment:

1. Rheumatic sicknesses (rheumatic polyarthritis, muscular and cardiac rheumatism).

2. Infectious polyarthritis of unspecific origin.

3. Deformed spondylitis-deformans.

4. Affections of the peripheral nervous system (radiculitis, lumbo-sacral inflammation of the sciatic, femoral, facial nerves, intercostal polyneuritis, neuralgias, etc.).

5. Trophic and sore ulcers, "slow granulation."

6. The surgical sicknesses of vessels (thrombosis, phlebitis without purulent process, endoarteriosclerosis, endarteritis, arteriosclerosis of the vessels of the extremities).

7. Infiltrated inflammatories (without pus).

8. Bronchial asthma.

9. Migraine.

10. Hypertonic sicknesses of 1st or 2nd degree.

11. Iritis and iridocyclitis, as well as thyrotoxicosis of 1st or 2nd degree.

One must not forget, that in certain sicknesses, bee-venom cannot be used in cases in which the organism of the patient has acquired an allergic hypersensitivity to bee-venom; also, in the following cases bee-venom must not be used: tuberculosis, venereal diseases, certain phychical sicknesses, hepatitis, nephritis, acute infectious sicknesses, acute purulent processes, insufficiency of the cardio-vascular system and serious exhaustion of the organism. Certain physicians advise against the use of bee-venom in the case of pregnant women and diabetes. . . .

Finally it is necessary to draw attention to the most important peculiarity of the therapeutic action of bee-venom—the re-adaptation of the organism's reactivity, i.e., the awakening of its defense-forces, immobilized by the disease. Thus, the organism begins to respond better to other therapeutic means. Only for this reason, does treatment with bee-venom combine well with other therapeutic methods.

It would be in error to place on the same footing, hormone-therapy and bee-venom treatment. The use of hormones gives a much faster and intensive effect, but this is temporary (of short duration), and is accompanied by secretions of corresponding glands. Venom, on the contrary, in stimulating the glands through reflex stirs them up for a longer time, but not in such a rapid way. . . . Probably the secretion of hormones is only a link in the complex chain of adaption and the defense process, while venom with its quality of a natural stimulant provokes the whole chain of processes.

CONCLUSION

The analysis of the physiological action of bee-venom, done in the light of data concerning the evolution of bees, has permitted us to draw some conclusions having, as it appears to us, not only biological value but also a certain medical value. The property of bee-venom to stimulate the defense-forces of the organism, its neurotoxic action and its gangliolytic effect in particular are of equal importance. These aspects of the action of bee-venom on the organism permit us to set forth a new explanation of the following phenomena, which are so important: the therapeutic effect of bee-venom, the complex syndrome of envenomation and finally the phenomenon of the immunity of bee-keepers.

1. We believe that the therapeutic action of bee-venom depends on the fact that the latter, being a natural specific stimulant in mobilizing the defense-forces of the organism, is capable of provoking, even in small amounts, a general, nonspecific reaction, such as a protective inhibition in the superior zones of the ganglions and the augmentation of internal secretions of the adrenal system. Venom provokes a series of active defense-reflexes. This reaction, which constitutes the general foundation of the therapeutic action of bee-venom, is the consequence of the evolution of the reciprocal action of the bees and mammifers during millions of years. Its development can explain the therapeutic effect of venom in rheumatism, allergies and other diseases, where the use of cortisone and of ACTH is indicated. The capacity of venom to block the transmission of excitations in the sympathetic ganglions has an equal therapeutic action. This allows us to understand the positive action of venom in arterial hypertension and obliterative endarteritis.

2. The hypothesis presented permits us to give a rational explanation and to make a classification of the symptoms of envenomation by bee-venom. Up to now, one has placed symptoms which have a different biological significance in the same category. . . . It is indispensable that one makes a distinction between the symptoms, which are caused by the destruction either of organs or of cells or of biochemical systems, and the phenomena, which constitute the defense reaction of the organism. All these symptoms must be considered in relation to their function and their reciprocal development; this should aid the clinicians in elaborating rational treatment methods of envenomation by bee-venom.

3. Finally, we see the possibility of considering [from] a new angle
. . . the phenomenon of immunity in bee-keepers, whose nature up
to now, has remained unknown. All the attempts to discover, in the
blood of bee-keepers or of animals immunized to bee-venom, specific antitoxins against the active principle of this venom, have
been in vain. We can consider the reduced sensibility (immunity)
of bee-keepers as a consequence of an increase in resistance to the
venom, which is the result of adaption, or more precisely of the
transition towards the stage of resistance of the general syndrome
of adaption.

If this hypothesis allows us to give the same explanation to
phenomena so far removed from each other, we are assured of
being on the right path and can hope to collaborate, by our work,
the efficacious use of bee-venom in medical practice and . . . the
development of a new branch of bee-keeping, which will have as its
only goal to serve the requirements of contemporary medicine.

The biggest damn spider I'd ever seen was crawling across
my bubble. I fetched my can of Raid, which I keep up forward
to shoot down flying mischief makers before they panic me
into an oncoming car. I put the Raid back after it had done its
work.

Hoooeee, what's that? Those lights are coming to get me. I
should have asked Ed Honl if I could sleep with his bees.
They're going to git me. Sure enough they're going to git me.

"Well, I was looking for a rest area and it got late and I just
pulled off the road. OK, Officer, I'll get out of here if I'm upsetting anybody. Yes, I've got identification." I handed him my
driver's license.

"You can talk to the owner while I check this out."

"I'm sorry if I disturbed you. I just saw this open field. I was
tired, so I thought I'd just pull off. I'll get out of here if I'm
bothering anybody."

"I was driving to the house and I saw your van out here. I
didn't know what you were up to, so I went and got the sheriff
here. You know you can't be too careful nowadays. A deputy
was shot dead by some kid from Georgia the other night."

"Yes, I understand that, and I don't want to infringe on your
property. I'll git on down the road. I'm doing some research on

bees and I was over talking with Ed Honl in Winthrop. Guess I stayed later than I should have."

The sheriff came back with my license.

"You're clean as a whistle as far as Minnesota's concerned."

"That's a relief," I mumbled. I always mumble.

"Look, you stay here as long as you want. If anybody bothers you just tell them the owner said it was OK. My name is Roger Hargish. Just tell them I said it was OK."

The guys from Stillwater Jail didn't get me, and the coon hunters didn't eat me. I took a tablespoon of honey and slept long and well, although lightning and rain played heavily on my skylight.

Mr. Joe Niehaus wasn't on my list of beekeepers. I just happened down his road one dark afternoon and spotted a few hives under the overhang of the barn. I passed by, drove a mile or two, and came back.

Mr. Niehaus was finishing up the last day at the legislature, and Mrs. Niehaus couldn't have been more cordial.

"Do you use honey for anything besides eating?"

"We use honey for everything—on our cereal, I bake with it. My husband used to have arthritis. It got so he couldn't lift up his arm to shave no more. And he started using honey for everything and the arthritis went away."

"Do you think it was the honey or getting stung?"

"I think it had a lot to do with the honey."

We had a good visit. Mr. and Mrs. Niehaus have seven children and twenty-two grandchildren. We talked about them a bit and then about what to do when a tornado comes. The radio had been broadcasting warnings all afternoon. Mrs. Niehaus is a nice lady.

Dave Sundenberg said, "I had an aunt who had diabetes, and honey was the only sweet that she could use."

"I'm glad to hear you say that. The doctor said she could use it?"

"She used it. I don't know how long she had diabetes, but it was ever since I had known her."

"Did she just take a small amount each day or eat it as she wished?"

"I couldn't exactly say, but I know she ate honey; she ate honey with the diabetes and didn't have any ill effects. It must not have affected her because she died of other causes."

"She didn't go into insulin shock?"

"No, no. It was something else. But I know she used honey all the time. I don't know if any doctor would recommend honey. But I know other diabetics who have used honey."

I explained that I wanted to include this use in my book and that I would like an American medical reference permitting its use.

Dave said, "Well, it's too bad Aunt Shopie's not still alive so you could get it right from the horse's mouth, so to speak."

"You don't know how to get in touch with her?"

"No, not anymore."

From N. Ioyrish's *Bees and People:*

The Moscow doctor A. Davydov described in 1915 how he had used honey with success in treating diabetics. After giving eight patients honey he concluded that "honey can be very useful in treating sugar diabetes in many cases: (1) as a tasty substance; (2) as a nutritious addition to the diabetic diet since there is almost no desire, when it is taken, for other sweet things not permitted in the illness; (3) as a means of preventing acetonaemia, for which sugar always has to be prescribed, so upsetting the diet; (4) as a sugar that not only does not increase excretion of glucose but even greatly reduces it."

And from Texas Dr. Joe Nichols's book:

I tell the diabetic to use unrefined salt, natural cold pressed oils, whole grain cereals and honey that has not been pasteurized. Even a diabetic can eat small quantities of natural honey.

Mind you, I am not suggesting that diabetics climb right into the honeypot. I have included this material so that diabetics and people who have glycemia may look into the possibilities of using honey.

The most beautiful farmland I've ever seen was in Minnesota in May of 1977. Land of newly plowed rich black soil rolling up to the horizon and capped by mature, new-green-leaved basswood trees silhouetted against dark storm clouds.

The farmhouses, set a quarter of a mile or more back from the road, were well designed and maintained with considerable pride. Ponds and small lakes fed the land and vice versa.

Those of you who worry that your love affair with America is flagging, take a slow motor trip up through central Minnesota and down through central Wisconsin during May. It will rejuvenate your soul, your hope, and your faith.

In my travels visiting with beekeepers I had run across a curious phenomenon. Many of the offspring of beekeepers are allergic to bee venom. This hypersensitivity probably can be explained in genetic terms. But even more curious is the high incidence of allergies among beekeepers' spouses. I refer to hypersensitivity that developed only after the marriage.

The national average for true bee venom allergies is 2.0 percent of the total population. There are no statistics available, but in my rough estimation 15 percent of the families I called on had either a child or a wife who was hypersensitive.

I did not intend to include this subject matter in this book because I did not think it germaine to the general topic. However, the last three beekeeping families I called on were intimately involved with venom allergies. And because of the wonderful reception given me by beekeeping families all across the country, I feel it incumbent on me to spread the word about Dr. Mary Lovelace's work.

I have focused your attention on Dr. Lovelace for two reasons. Many beekeepers will read this book and know where to get certain help. And maybe some benefactor will make the necessary funds available so that the necessary form can be followed and Dr. Lovelace's procedures accepted by the FDA.

The interview that prompted this decision took place in North Dakota.

"We had a daughter who died about three years ago from bee stings. What the doctor had done was use this ground-up-bee serum and she went through a series of shots. When it was all over, everything was OK, we were told. But the doctor didn't say anything about booster shots. We didn't know anything about it. I could blame the doctors for not being more concerned. She was down in Oklahoma and got a few stings with absolutely no problem. About three weeks after that we were up here and she got stung on the foot, had a severe anaphylactic reaction, and suffocated. So we figure she was protected for a few stings, but each sting she got, she was less protected and she had no protection when she got her last sting."

"Dr. Lovelace told me about this sort of thing happening with the ground-up-bee serum," I said. "She says that with the method she uses this doesn't happen. Once you're immunized, you have to be checked once a year. Rarely, you may have to get a booster, but generally speaking one series of shots is enough." I knew this information was small comfort to these parents.

This interview left me in a sludge of gloom.

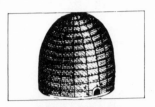

SIXTEEN

Dr. E.V. McCollum, formerly Professor of Chemical Hygiene, School of Hygiene and Public Health, Johns Hopkins University, addressed the Northern Ohio Dental Association's seventieth anniversary and said that "the American people ought to be ashamed in permitting two atrocities to be put over on them." He referred in particular to white flour and refined sugar. McCollum said that he "sometimes wondered which of the two evils is greater." That was more than forty years ago.

More than twenty years ago Dr. William Coda Martin had this to say about refined sugar:

What is left consists of pure, refined carbohydrates. The body cannot utilize this refined starch and carbohydrate unless the depleted proteins, vitamins, and minerals are present. Nature supplies these elements in each plant in quantities sufficient to metabolize the carbohydrate in that particular plant. There is no excess for other added carbohydrates. Incomplete carbohydrate metabolism results in the formation of "toxic metabolites" such as pyruvic acid and abnormal sugars containing 5 carbon atoms. Pyruvic acid accumulates in the brain and nervous system and the abnormal sugars in the red blood cells. These toxic metabolites interfere with the respiration of the cells. They cannot get sufficient oxygen to survive and function normally. In time some of the cells die. This interferes with the function of a part of the body and is the beginning of degenerative disease. With over 50 percent of our diet today composed of these refined carbohydrates (refined sugar, white flour, polished rice, macaroni, and most breakfast cereals), does it require a million dollars for research to find out why this generation is developing more and more degenerative diseases?

In 1975, Dr. Joe Nichols wrote in *Please, Doctor, Do Something:*

White sugar fits in perfectly with white rice and white bread. They are buddies. White sugar is the worst food in the American diet. I have stated innumerable times, "It is so sorry that not even a worm will eat it." The fact is that white sugar is one of our most dangerous food items in this country.

Refined sugar is 99.9 percent pure, so they say.

Not so honey. Honey has all this stuff in it: fructose (38 percent); dextrose (31 percent); sucrose (1 percent); vitamins B_1, B_2, B_6, and C; calcium; iron; phosphorus; copper; manganese; potassium; sodium; magnesium; sulfur; chlorine; and these known enzymes—invertase, diatase, catalase, inulase, and phosphatase.

What's the good of all this? I wish I could quote from an American source, but the American medical establishment seems to feel that the *only* difference between refined sugar and honey is that honey is 15 percent sweeter. This quote is taken from a paper by S. Mladenov, a Bulgarian, presented to the International Symposium on Apitherapy in Madrid in 1974:

At present we have a rich experimental and clinic material, obtained after the successful application of apitherapy at the Balneary sanatorium of Kinstendil to over 15,000 patients suffering especially from respiratory diseases. At the same time we have studied the effects of this therapy on the other organs and systems of the patients.

1. Internal application, oral administration.

DOSAGE: daily, 1–2 g per kg-weight. In the case of the respiratory affections one recommends honey retained in the mouth cavity, six times a day. In the case of gastric-intestinal, kidney, and liver diseases, and neuroses—we recommend honey dissolved in warm water, three times before the main meals, or at three hours after meals, according to the nature of the disease.

2. AEROSOL INHALATIONS. A solution of 20–30% honey in distilled water or saline solution which vaporizes in particles with the dimensions of 5–50 microns, is inhaled for 20 minutes, once or twice a day. This form of treatment is applied in the case of the diseases with inflammatory character and of allergies of the breathing apparatus.

3. LOCAL APPLICATIONS. It is used in case of rhinitis, pharyngitis, sinusitis, laryngitis, colpitis, atrophic and suppurative wounds.

4. ELECTROPHORESIS WITH 30% HONEY SOLUTION. It is used in cases of rhinitis, sinusitis, bronchitis, colpitis, trichomoniasis, parametritis, adnexitis. It lasts for 15–30 minutes, once a day (5–20 mA).

5. THROAT WASHES AND LAVEMENTS WITH 30% HONEY SOLUTION. In cases of stomatitis, pharyngitis, laryngitis, colpitis: two–four times a day.
The effects of the therapy over the body are the following:

a. Immunobiological: it increases the resistance of the body.
b. Antibacterial.
c. Antiinflammatory.
d. Regenerating: it regenerates the affected cells and tissues.
e. Expectorant: it dilutes the bronchial secretions, improves the functions of the bronchi epithelium as well as their peristaltic waves.

6. Analgesic and sedative: it diminishes the pain in the affected area; it improves sleep.

7. Hyposensitiser.

In the case of affections of the respiratory system—rhinitis, sinusitis, pharyngitis, laryngitis, tracheitis, bronchitis, asthmatic bronchitis—in 88% of the cases one obtains a permanent therapeutic effect. The treatments last in general for 20 days, consisting of two aerosol inhalations per day with the prescribed honey dose.

In cases of rhinitis, sinusitis, pharyngitis, and laryngitis one also uses local applications in the nostrils. When needed, the treatment may be repeated several times.

The fuel consumption of a flying bee is about 7 million miles to a gallon of honey. In providing one surplus pound of honey for the "robbers," the colony must consume about eight pounds to keep itself going. The foraging has probably covered a total flight path equal to three orbits around the earth at a fuel consumption of about an ounce of honey for each orbit. That's good mileage.

In *Apitherapy Today,* Harnaj and coauthors describe how bees make honey:

To understand the process by which nectar is transformed into honey, let us follow the collecting bee: in quest of nectar the bee alights on a flower. She explores it, eventually opening the corolla with her mandibles, and finds the nectariferous glands from which she will suck the nectar with her proboscis, to deposit it for the duration of transport in her crop. The processing of honey in the bee's inner laboratory starts from this moment. By the direct agency of the bee, the nectar will change completely its consistency and its compositional structure.

During the return flight, part of the water contained in nectar is eliminated through the walls of the crop. Stimulated by the pressure of nectar in the crop, part of the bee's glands start secreting several specific ferments which influence the chemical and biochemical transformation process of nectar.

Once back in the hive, the collecting bee is met by a young bee—which, in the first days of life, is called the "the hive bee," because the division of labour compels her to fulfill several functions inside the hive—and delivers to the latter the nectar collected, to be deposited in honeycombs cells.

Upon this occasion—being transferred from one bee to another, from one crop to another—the nectar receives new amounts of ferments, especially of invertin.

This nectar does not remain in the first cell it was deposited in. Another young bee comes and moves it so that it passes a great many times from crop to crop, from cell to cell, and each time the transformation process increases in intensity, till the nectar becomes honey. As a rule, these shiftings occur by night. During the storage of nectar in cells the surplus water, which is superfluous in the chemical process, is removed by the activity of ventilating bees, so that the concentration degree will correspond to the characteristics of mature honey. Bees have to collect 3 or 4 kg of nectar to obtain one kg of ripe (mature) honey.

When the bees begin to seal the cells, it means that the transformation process of nectar into honey is almost finished, and the honey is mature (when half the honeycomb is sealed). In this case, it contains about 20% water—the normal content in high-grade honey.

The average annual sugar consumption per person in the United States is 108 pounds. The average honey consumption per person is 1.5 pounds. I suggest that if these ratios were reversed the salubrious effect on Americans would be remarkable. Of course, there is nothing you personally can do to reverse these ratios. But you might consider the advisability of treating your own body more like a temple and less like a cauldron.

Whenever possible eat "raw" or "unpasteurized" or "uncooked" honey. Honey quite often granulates, and this makes it less salable to the general public. So packagers heat the honey to prevent this granulation, and then they run it through fine filters. This process kills the enzymes and removes the pollens, thereby considerably reducing the goodness of the honey. Always get raw, uncooked, or unpasteurized honey and don't worry about the cloudiness.

In the oldest written documents known—the clay slabs of Mesopotamian culture, dating as far back as 2700 BC—honey is mentioned as being used as a medicine. In 1970, surgeons Cavanagh, Beazley, and Ostapowicz had the courage to use and report on the beneficial effect of honey on wound healing. Can't we afford to learn everything there is to learn about the powers of honey and other bee products?

The U.S. Congress authorized a $100 million subsidy for the sugar growers in 1977.

Only recently have beekeepers been collecting pollen for their own consumption. This is probably why I discovered very few medicinal uses for pollen among the beekeepers I called on.

Here is a good synopsis, taken from *The People's Almanac:*

Pollen is the male germ seed of plants and flowers, and a single grain is invisible to the naked eye. It is gathered by bees, who collect it in sacs on their back legs and take it to the hive. There it is either formed into royal jelly—which is fed exclusively to the queen and which gives her her special powers—or it is combined with honey to make bee bread, which is the food of the drones and workers. Pollen has been mentioned in the ancient writings of Egypt, China, Greece, and Russia, and experiments are presently being conducted to determine how best it can be used to help humans, since it is proving to be an amazing food. It is free from added colors, chemicals, and preservatives and is the richest source yet revealed of minerals, vitamins, and amino acids. Pollen may be as much as 13% complete protein, and in detail, it contains large quantities of vitamins A, B, C, D, E, and K; plus rutin, lecithin, amines, nuclein, guanine, xanthine, hydrocarbons, and sterol. In fact, pollen is a complete food, with a built-in life force, and the only similar food that can be compared to it is yeast. Antibiotics are present naturally, and it can be stored without loss of vitality. In medicine, its uses are only just being discovered. Cernitin, a pollen extract, has been used successfully in the treatment of influenza, urinary disorders, and measles. Tests in France prove pollen has been instrumental in curing anemia in young children and chronic constipation in adults. It helps in the recovery from shock, and as a tonic and energy restorer, it has given a new lease on life to old men. In fact, its potential appears to be unlimited. Pollen is present in varying amounts in all honeys, and it can also be purchased in powder or tablet form.

What better inducement to use pollen can I offer you than the fact that it is the only food you can ingest which has every single element your blood requires to be healthy?

In Russia bees collect annually 200,000 tons of pollen. I don't know how much is collected in the United States, but wouldn't it be the cat's whiskers if the government made a concerted effort to get pollen into every schoolchild and old person in the United States?

Propolis (bee glue) and royal jelly have many remarkable

therapeutic qualities, but it is of small value to recount them here because these products, in a refined state, are not available in North America.

The U.S. government's attitude toward honey and other bee products can best be typified by the following story.

Dr. Jarvis's book *Folk Medicine* strongly advocates the use of vinegar and honey to cure many of our maladies. Honey retailers, quite naturally, offered this book for sale. Apparently it is against the law to sell a book recommending the medicinal value of a food product if that product is within fifty feet of the book.

So the U.S. marshals confiscated the inventories of a select number of honey retailers, and the matter went to federal court. The retailers' attorney pointed out, during the course of the trial, that the Bible favorably mentions bees, honey, and honeycomb sixty-eight times.

The judge ruled that the honey retailers could sell neither *Folk Medicine* nor the Bible within fifty feet of the honey products.

And so it goes.

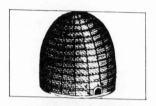

SEVENTEEN

BACK TO THE exciting saga of me and my stinging. By the time I returned to Victoria, British Columbia, there was no question that I had a mess of arthritis in my feet. I seemed to have trigger points in every foot joint. I also had a multitude of trigger points around both ankles.

It took only three or four stinging sessions to get rid of each of the trigger points in my feet. My feet became loose and freer. What I had long assumed were tight-fitting shoes were actually metatarsals jammed with arthritis. The ankles were harder to clear up and took a lot of dedicated stinging.

Charlie Mraz and Dr. Saine advised heavy doses of vitamins, particularly C. Because I thought I had an "allergy" to vitamin C, I had not been taking it. When I read about the neurosurgeon in Texas who cured his back problem with vitamin C, I decided to give it a whirl. It seemed to me I made dramatic improvement after that. And no matter how many stings I took I did not get a feeling of fatigue or lethargy after starting on the C.

Men, monkeys, and guinea pigs are the only mammals that cannot manufacture their own vitamin C. Science discovered in 1935 that arthritics have a subnormal supply of vitamin C. Bee venom seems to lower the vitamin C level further. Colonel Vick's later tests in monkeys indicate that as vitamin C increases so does the production of natural cortisone when bee venom is administered.

Government regulation requires that monkeys maintained by the government be fed 1,000 milligrams of vitamin C a day in order to keep them healthy. Based on relative body weight, our RDA (recommended daily allowance) would be 4,000 milligrams.

If I were taking BV now, I would use 4,000 milligrams of vitamin C in 500-milligram doses spread equally throughout the day. Toward the end of my treatment I took 3,000 milligrams, but I now believe 4,000 milligrams would be better.

I have stung my knees 502 times, my back 212, my hips 23, my left foot 483, and my right foot 506. This totals 1,726. I am convinced that had I, or the doctors, discovered early on that my knee problems were in my feet and ankles, and if I had taken vitamin C from the beginning, I would have rid myself of the arthritis more quickly.

The most stings I took at any one sitting were 104. I noticed a slight increase in heartbeat for an hour or so after that. The most pronounced general reaction I had, overall, was nausea in Tennessee after thirteen stings. I assumed that this was caused by the bee venom, but I am not certain.

I don't advocate taking as many as 104 stings at one time. I did it because I was anxious for some conclusive results. But as we know, if a good thing is good, more is not necessarily better.

Presumably you either have arthritis or someone close to you has it. You wouldn't have come along this far if you didn't think there was perhaps just a shred of truth in what I've been preaching.

The first and easiest step is to start eating honey as Messrs. Colson, Niehaus, and Waite do. Try it for a couple of months. Then perhaps you should try Mrs. Colson's honey and apple-cider vinegar treatment; or P.A. Yelverton's honey and Certo; or H. Lange's honey, Epsom salts, and lemon remedy.

Center Laboratory, Inc., of Long Island, now markets inject-able bee venom serum. The FDA has approved the use of bee venom for the desensitization of bee venom allergies.

Dr. Israeli Jaffe of New York Medical College was quoted in an interview in a national publication reporting on a new arthritis drug: "There's a clause in the FDA regulations which states that if a physician wants to prescribe an approved drug for an unapproved indication—because in his opinion there's nothing better—he may do so."

Of course, the trick is to find a physician cut from the same cloth as Drs. Carey and Sanders.

I believe that if your arthritis is curable, Dr. Joseph Saine in Montreal is the one who can cure it. He injects bee venom serum hypodermically or by ionization if the patient is highly sensitive or allergic.

If you find that treatment in Europe would be more conve-nient, write to:

> Heinrich Mack Nachfolger
> Chemisch-Pharmazeutische Fabrik
> Postfach 140
> D-7918 Illertissen/Bayern
> West Germany

and ask them to give you a list of the doctors and clinics who use their product, Forapin, in the countries in which you are interested. Bulgaria has had excellent results using a bee venom ointment with ultrasound.

You can wait for the medical profession in the United States to offer you the freedom of decision—whether you wish gold salts, cortisone, surgery, or bee venom. On May 25, 1977, the Food and Drug Administration advised that no investigational new drug application for the experimental testing of bee venom on arthritics had been filed with them. This means that availability of serum and governmental approval of the tech-nique are nowhere in sight. However, this could change quickly if enough pressure were exerted.

If you want to sting yourself, this is extremely important: Go to a doctor and be tested for sensitivity to bee venom. It's a very simple procedure. You may have been stung frequently when young and not been seriously bothered. However, sensitivities can later develop, and it would be prudent to take this precaution.

Also keep this in mind: While it sometimes happens, it is not usual that one or two stings will cure you. In fairness to yourself, you must decide that you are going to give it a good shot and not become discouraged if you don't have early success.

Be sure you have a good, constant source of bees. Running out of bees is disappointing. Remember that the beekeeper cannot get bees when the weather is cold, and he quite likely won't mess with the bees when it is cloudy or rainy because then they are much ill-disposed. Obviously, in most parts of the States it would be well to start your program in the spring. Most beekeepers will be happy to give you the bees. But offer them a couple of bucks anyway. The bees are going to be worth far more to you.

Get two one-gallon pickle or mayonnaise jars from your favorite restaurateur and be sure they are sparkling clean. A one-gallon jar will hold 500 bees easily. The reason for two jars is that you'll want to move the bees from one jar to the other in order to keep them clean. Bees get depressed and lethargic around dirt, and we must keep the ladies happy.

Take some paper toweling, fold it over, and lay a half dozen thicknesses on the bottom of the jar. Fill a jar cap with honey, put a swatch of nylon screening over this, and tape the screening to one side of the cap to keep it from shifting around. Put this cap on the paper toweling. The ladies can then partake of the honey without getting stuck and done in by it. Don't feed them anything else or water them. The only thing they like better than honey in a cap is honey in a comb, but that's so hard to come by that I didn't suggest it.

Next, put in a cardboard cylinder, such as you get from a roll of paper towels. This should be long enough so that it rests on an angle against where the jar curves to the opening. Punch some holes in the cover for air and you're in business.

Give the ladies light. Darkness quiets them down, but too much of it makes them morose. The ladies will cluster in and on the cone, especially at night. Night is a good time to transfer them to a second jar—after the first is dirty. Simply lift the cylinder gently with your medical tweezers and lower it into the second jar. A few bees will remain behind and they can be transferred individually with your tweezers. Grab them gently by the middle part of their bodies.

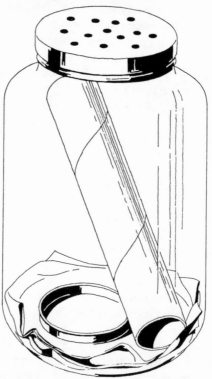

Sometimes you may have to transfer them every three or four days. On the other hand, I've gone ten days without having to change and clean jars. Why, I don't know.

Don't fret about the bees stinging you accidently. In ten months of working with the ladies I've never been stung accidently. If in securing a bee, one or more slip out of the jar, don't panic or worry. They will fly straight to a light source—a window or a lamp—and usually rest easy. You can then pick them off at your leisure. Bear in mind that they generally will not sting unless you've secured them or are molesting the hive.

I would advise having two pairs of long medical (or dental) tweezers. You will be reaching down into the jar to get a hold on the head or the thorax (the middle part of the bee, between the head and the tail). But it doesn't always work that way—you might grab her by the legs, wings, abdomen, etc. In that case you can use the second pair of tweezers to get her in a better position.

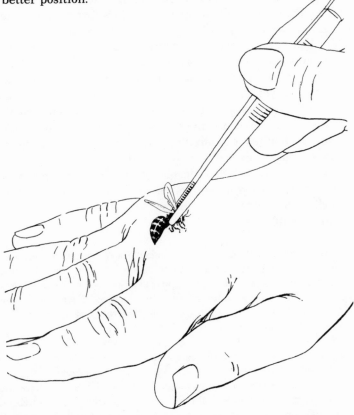

If you're concerned about the pain of the sting, this is very important. Put a plastic glass filled with water in the freezer and make a nice solid lump of ice. Get yourself all set up with the cap of the jar loosened, your tweezers at the ready, and then put the ice on the area you are going to sting. Hold the ice there until you can't feel the cold anymore and then apply the sting. If you do this, I think I can assure you that you will hardly know you've been stung. The bee venom itself has a numbing effect, and subsequent stings will carry less clout. I found that in stinging my ankle a hundred times at a sitting, I needed the cold treatment for only four stings, if they were strategically placed around the ankle. However, particularly in the beginning, numb all spots with ice before applying the sting. Martyrdom is not the purpose of the exercise.

The bee will not always quickly dislodge her stinger in your flesh and sometimes you may have to give her a little punch in the back. (Folklore has it that bees will not sting a dead person, so if you can't get the bees to sting you, further api-therapy is contraindicated.) Once the stinger is in you, remove the bee and allow the stinger to work itself in for about ten minutes. Then just squeeze the poison sac with the tweezers to get the last drop and remove the stinger.

What has just preceded was gleaned from my own personal experience. Let me quote from some material given me by Charlie Mraz, who is a beeman, not a doctor, but is pretty knowledgeable.

It appears that arthritics are usually not allergic to bee venom, and over the past 100 years in which bee venom has been used to treat arthritic patients, there does not appear to be a single case of a fatality recorded. This is a record few other drugs can boast. Even aspirin, the mildest of the drugs commonly used for the relief of arthritis, does have fatalities to its record.

If a person is allergic to stings, he usually knows he is allergic because of a previous experience that developed the sensitivity. There is also some misunderstanding as to what is an allergic reaction. In a true allergic reaction, the whole body reacts, no matter where the person is stung. The eyes will swell and water, there will be itching of scalp, palms of the hands, and soles of the feet. The whole body will break out in red blotches. Up to this stage, it is not particularly danger-ous, and a person will usually respond quickly to antihistamines and Adrenalin. Beyond this state there can be a drop of blood pressure and difficulty in breathing, which is a dangerous condition and needs treatment immediately with Adrenalin injections and antihistamine. There are methods for desensitizing for such conditions.

A person is not allergic if the sting produces a swelling only in the area in which the sting is applied, and it does not matter how large the swelling is. Sometimes a person getting a sting on the knee will swell from the ankle to the hips. This is not an allergic reaction if the reaction is confined to the sting area, no matter how large. In fact, such reactions produce the best therapeutic results.

If an arthritic has never been stung or never has experienced an allergic reaction to insect stings, chances are he is not allergic. In my own experience of forty years, I have not seen a serious case of allergy in a person being treated for rheumatic diseases. Occasionally, during a course of treatment, a person will show some primary allergic reactions, but a reduction in the venom with a gradual increase will usually produce a resistance to bee venom. This experience is shared by most of the doctors that have used bee venom therapy for many years. Danger of an allergic reaction appears to be a minor problem with arthritics. . . .

Before any therapy is started, the person must first be tested for any possible allergic reaction. [Emphasis added.] This is done by applying a sting and then removing it instantly, after being assured that there is no history of allergy. Wait for fifteen minutes or half an hour and if there is no allergic reaction in this time, there is no allergic problem. In half an hour another sting can be applied and this also removed quickly. This is usually enough for the first treatment.

After that the serious business of therapy can be started. If the arthritis is of an acute type, of short duration, no damage to the joints and only a few local points involved, the treatment is usually only of short duration and only a few stings are necessary. Sometimes a local condition will clear up with only one sting, but normally a series of treatments is required. The first day, start with just the two test stings and continue every day for about a week with two to four stings each day, depending on the severity of the arthritis.

While bee venom has systemic as well as a local reaction, the best results are found by treating the trigger points. These trigger points are over the part of the body where arthritis is involved. Basically, arthritis of the upper part of the body stems from the upper spine, and arthritis of the lower part of the body from the lower spine. For this reason, it is a good idea to use the spine area as a base of operations. Treat the spine area first. Then work down from the spine toward the extremities: the shoulders, neck, elbows, wrists, hands, and so on. From the lower spine, work toward the hips, knees, and ankles, where trigger points are found.

With experience, one can soon find out how many stings he can take without too much discomfort. At first, the stings may produce very little pain, but as the treatment is continued, the body will again be more sensitive to pain as the arthritic symptoms leave the areas. This is a good sign that there is improvement in the condition. If the arthritic condition is severe, after the first week of two to four stings each day, treat every other day using more stings as needed. It may be necessary to give ten to twenty stings with each treatment for bad cases. It must be remembered, in serious cases of joint damage, no type of treatment can make new joints or tissue. In such cases, one can only expect to get relief of pain and to stop the progress of the disease.

A course of treatment usually lasts from four to eight weeks, with treatments every other day. The stings should be applied to different areas each time so as not to treat an area that is still swollen.

Usually when treatments are first started, there is very little or no swelling. Then as treatment is continued, the areas will begin to swell much more, with redness and itching of the areas treated. Sometimes during this stage, the patient will feel worse—more pain and pain in areas never before affected. There may be nausea and a feeling of discouragement. It is important to remember this is a good sign that the treatment is working and treatment must be continued. The number of stings can be reduced, if desired. It appears that the cause of this reaction is the purging of toxins from the body by the stimulation of the biotic processes of the body. It follows the classical Hans Selye syndrome of the stages of reaction and then the stage of resistance. Soon after this, the stings will no longer swell and a person becomes "immune," just as a beekeeper becomes immune after working with bees a long time. When one reaches this "immune stage," the first course of treatment can be terminated.

At this point a person will usually find his condition much improved. No more treatment is necessary for another month or two, and if there is no return of the arthritic symptoms, there is no longer need of any further treatments for a period of perhaps several years or as long as twenty years or more. However, if after a "rest period" of a month or two, there are still arthritic symptoms, another course of treatments can be followed, starting with one sting and building up as with the first course. However, with subsequent courses, the treatments are usually more effective and with quicker results so that a shorter course of treatments will suffice. In very bad cases, three or more courses of treatments may be necessary covering a period of two years or more. However, in the usual cases where there is little or no joint damage, a few weeks of treatment will suffice.

In addition to the stinging, don't eat *any* refined sugar and eliminate bleached white flour as much as possible. Russian therapists recommend two to three ounces of *raw* honey a day. Not only does this tend to eliminate poisons from your body and act as a sedative, it also seems to have antiarthritic properties. Take a lot of vitamins, particularly B_1 and C, and pollen. And no booze. Keep a journal. Record the number of stings, locations, focal and general reactions.

So much for you. You can accept or reject this "home remedy." But how about the big picture? How long, if ever, will it be before the medical profession in the United States proves whether Terc, Beck, Broadman, Carey, Guyton, Sanders, Saine, and thousands of former arthritics are right or wrong?

I don't expect this book will provoke any action from the medical establishment except perhaps cries of quackery. This is OK. But I do hope the book will provoke you to do this:

1. Write to your congressman and both senators urging them to read the article "Arthritis and Bees" in the May 19, 1974, *Washington Post,* pp. C1 and C5.

2. Ask them to answer these questions after they've had a chance to read this article:

a. Why can't the people who are interested in bee venom research get cooperation from the drug companies?
b. Why couldn't funding be found for "five good clinical labs spending more than $100,000 each for two years with [arthritic] patients tested toward the end of these studies"?
c. Why doesn't Congress open an inquiry into the whole field of bee venom and arthritis, heart disease, and cancer?

And while you're in a writing mood, write to:

The Arthritis Foundation
3400 Peachtree Road N.E.
Atlanta, Georgia 30326

Point out that you are not going to make any further contributions until the foundation agrees "to set aside funds contributed which are specifically designated for bee venom research," as Dr. Sisk promised to do, according to the May 19, 1974, *Washington Post* article.

If enough of you write the above letters, we'll get some action. If you believe there is some substance in what you've read, and you do nothing, shame on you.

Perhaps you have some big bucks and an itch to do something really worthwhile, while you're still alive and before the lawyers and the IRS get to scrapping over the treasure you may leave behind. Set up a foundation to explore, and test in accordance with the FDA's game rules, *all* the beehive products. If you are so inclined, ferreting out, exposing, and/or confirming just some of the claims made herein will take you all over the world and introduce you to some fascinating people and a captivating miniculture, a swarm of bees.

You might call it the "Apitherapy Medical Association." Doesn't that have an agreeable ring? It will probably be the most important thing you'll ever do.

Glenn Warren has done such a thing. When he was twelve he got arthritis and has suffered ever since. When he and Mrs. Warren were married, he was five inches taller than she. He is now five inches shorter. He was general manager of General Electric's turbine division and a vice-president. God knows what he would have become if he hadn't had this distraction. He has enormous intellect, compassion, and patience. He established the tax-exempt Glenn Warren Foundation to help solve the arthritis mystery. He has poured thousands of dollars and hours into it, although he realizes it is too late to help himself. His foundation has financed the work Dr. Weissmann did on rats, Colonel Vick's work on dogs and monkeys, Dr. Benton's work proving bee venom was not toxic, Shipman's work on arthritic horses, and much more. But perhaps most exciting of all, as a result of the Warren Foundation's funding, Colonel Vick and his associates have developed a bee venom ointment using cocoa butter as the vehicle. Early results indicate that it is just as effective as the live bee sting and it goes on and feels like hand lotion. What a joyful breakthrough.

You read in the 1974 *Washington Post* article of the interest and offers to help the Warren Foundation by members of various institutions. These offers were made predicated on Warren's establishing a certain protocol for testing on people. With the protocol ready, a prestigious rheumatologist can submit the forms requesting the required $200,000 from the government to prove whether or not bee venom works. The protocol has been ready for three years, and Warren is still waiting for the promised help. He's eighty years old now.

So, folks, raise hell with your congressman and send some bucks to:

The Glenn B. & Gertrude P. Warren Foundation, Inc.
1361 Myron Street
Schenectady, New York 12309

It's tax deductible, and if enough of you send money the clinical tests can be conducted without waiting for a prestigious rheumatologist to "mail in the coupons."

As you may have gathered, the mammoth pharmaceutical corporations are apparently not too interested in proving bee venom. Maybe just people will do it.

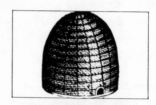

EIGHTEEN

THERE ARE approximately 50 million people in the United States who suffer with arthritis in varying degrees. You either have it or you don't. And if you don't, you don't worry about it because you know if you get it, it won't kill you, although the drugs might. And it's considered a disease of the elderly, although it isn't necessarily.

But cancer is something else again. Fear? Some people won't even say the word. According to the latest projections, one out of four people in the United States will get cancer, and one out of five will die from it. That's about 45 million people.

I guess that's really the reason I did all this traveling and research. The second beekeeper I met, William Matson, said that in twenty-five years he had never known a beekeeper to die of cancer. Extraordinary, absolutely extraordinary—and yet perhaps just a coincidence.

The third beekeeper I met (back in October 1976) was Clyde Wood, who had had Hodgkin's disease in 1935 and either the chiropractor or bee stings cured him. He's seventy-nine now. The AP news service carried an article on him in June 1977. Mr. Wood got calls from twenty-two people asking how he did it. Mr. Wood assumed they were all people who were afflicted with Hodgkin's disease.

Ironically, the first beekeeper I spoke with, Charlie Mraz, perhaps knows more about this subject than most anybody else in the United States. In a paper delivered to the Second Symposium on Apitherapy in Bucharest in 1976, Charlie said: "I personally know of cases where exposure to apitherapy has cured cases of cancer, such as breast cancer, cancer of the lip, leukemia, Hodgkin's disease, head tumor, etc." I believe if I discovered I had cancer, Charlie would be the first one I'd call.

Every professional beekeeper and entomologist I met, I asked: "Did you ever know a professional beekeeper to die of cancer?" I got so many negative answers that it occurred to me that maybe it was a loaded question because of the phraseology. So I changed the question to: "How many beekeepers do you know who have died of cancer?" These men generally were fifty to seventy years old, had been beekeepers for twenty-five to fifty years and active in their field. They knew beemen all across the country. I found three who had died of cancer. One of those contracted cancer after falling out of a tree and injuring his head badly. Another drank a good deal.

But this is hardly convincing evidence and from a zealous swagman, buzzing around the country in a van, taking random samplings.

Dr. W. Schweisheimer, in the September 1967 issue of *Gleanings in Bee Culture,* had this to say:

A strange observation some 20 years ago had been made by the Berlin Cancer Institute. Its scientists and doctors had never seen a beekeeper who was suffering from cancer.

For many years they had turned their attention to this particular problem. Another discovery they made was that they never saw a beekeeper who was suffering from gout. This, however, is an observation which has been described frequently and which dates back a good many centuries. It has been repeated time and again.

A later publication by Drs. Gunther Anton and Karl August Forester in Berlin has also stated that fewer beekeepers have suffered from cancer than the average of the population. They found among 19,026 members of beekeeping societies in Germany 0.36 in 1,000 (or about 1 among 3,000) cancer patients. . . .

The belief that beekeepers are relatively immune to cancer, as well as the widespread opinion that members of this profession exhibit unusual resistance to rheumatic diseases, seem to Prof. Cramer to be indication of a non-specific increase in immunity. This means that the higher resistance of the beekeeper's body does protect him against various diseases, not only against cancer or against gout or rheumatism. The increased resistance of the beekeeper's body may apply with equal effectiveness to bacterial diseases as to malignant growths (cancer).

That's better, but still fragmentary and perhaps too conjectural. Let me hang this on you. It's the last piece of research material of any sort that I've been able to get for this book. And I got it just several days ago from Clyde Wood.

In the New York Cancer Research Institute, Inc., *Annual Report,* we find the following:

Since acute inflammation seems to be one of the body's important defenses not only against infections, but against cancer, how cautious should we be in using the many new anti-inflammatory drugs, such as the anti-histamines, and more especially cortisone and its derivatives? Why do beekeepers have the lowest incidence of cancer? Perhaps it is because they are continually receiving injections of bee venom—i.e., bee stings, which cause an acute inflammatory reaction, liberating histamine which then activates the reticuloendothelial system—another important defense mechanism against cancer.

Hot damn, now that's more like it! "Why do beekeepers have the lowest incidence of cancer?" asks the New York Cancer Research Institute.

That was the annual report for *1965.* Aren't there enough funds in cancer research to find out *precisely why* beekeepers have the lowest incidence of cancer? If they learn that, won't they learn how to immunize everyone? Is the answer bee venom inoculations? Or is this too simple a solution?

Write to your congressmen and ask why the people weren't

told about this phenomenon. Ask them to find out what else cancer research scientists know about bee venom and cancer. If I were you, I would not be quieted until I had some very satisfying answers or strong commitments to get some very satisfying answers. Do it. Our lives may depend on it.

You have read in the previous pages of the stimulating effect bee venom has on the pituitary-adrenal system—causing it to generate higher outputs of adrenocortical steroids.

Here are some quotes, *out of context,* taken from the 1969 Drug Efficacy Study to the Commissioner of Food and Drugs, National Academy of Sciences. Remember this is the manufactured drug, not the natural product. The natural product could be more effective:

Adrenocortical steroids are temporarily useful in the palliative management of certain forms of neoplastic disease. . . .

The exact mechanism of action of adrenocortical steroids on neoplastic cells is not known. They inhibit the growth of mesenchymal cells and produce pyknosis and disintegration of lymphocytes. This may explain the favorable effect of these components on acute lymphoblastic leukemia, lymphosarcoma and other related lymphomas.

Is that why Clyde Wood, beekeeper, defeated Hodgkin's disease?

William Shipman, a biochemist with the navy in San Diego, was kind enough to allow me to rummage through two file drawers he has on bee venom research. The last folder in the file revealed a quote by Shipman in the Foundation for Nutrition and Stress *Research Bulletin,* March 1969:

The most exciting discovery from the horse work done for the Warren Foundation was a side experiment performed on another horse with a sidebone growth. His owner tried to save him earlier by having the nerves in his leg cut to relieve the pain of the side bone. After one operation a neuroma formed. A second operation was performed to remove the tumor but the neuroma formed a second time. We then injected bee venom weekly into the neuroma and found that it started to shrink. After four injections it was gone.

Because of the successful treatment of the neuroma and of the findings made with the bee venom experiments on bone marrow stem cells, Leonard Cole and I performed some experiments to assess the possible effect of BV on Leukemia. We found a powerful in vitro effect and alimental system effect. These studies are still in progress and a valid interpretation of the results is not possible at this time. However it can be said that a systemic effect does exist although its extent and value are undetermined.

Those tests were made at the naval laboratory in San Francisco. The funding ended, the laboratory closed, Leonard Cole died, and so the leukemia work ended.

Dr. Carey told me the following story about Charlie Mraz:

"One of the most recent was an amazing thing. A man had an eye that was protruding, pushed out by a tumor growing inside his skull and on the side of his head near his temple. This was causing the eye to popeye as it were, bug out. Evidently a man in his middle age. He went to one of the big cancer institutes, and they wouldn't touch it with X rays or chemotherapy because that particular area was not a good place to try it. So he was desperate, of course. They always are in these cases.

"He asked Charlie if bee stings would help. Well, everybody will ask you, 'Will it help this; will it help that?'

"So Charlie says, 'What do you have to lose?' It was the only answer he could give. He didn't know what it would do.

"Well, the man started to put bees on, and in a very short time the lump began to recede and the eye went back into place. The man subsequently bought an automobile agency in Jamaica, New York, is in business, working, and in good health."

What does all this prove?

Nothing.

But every single day that I read a newspaper, turn on the radio, or talk with a friend, I am confronted with the sinister specter of cancer. Billions have been spent without any definitive answers. Isn't there just a couple of million dollars in that moneybag to check the bee venom–cancer connection?

If there is something intrinsically evil about the honeybee, the Bible and I are unaware of it.

Well, here I write, on the west coast of Vancouver Island, parked on an old World War II military road that slips into the Pacific just a couple of feet away. We've been 32,818 miles together, and it has been the most rewarding experience of my life. Almost without exception, I have been handled royally. In addition to the people mentioned, there were dozens more who treated me handsomely. People such as Forrest Thomas in Vista, California; Mac Jenkins in Harrison, Arkansas; and Rando Hines in Cumberland Gap, Virginia. Splendid people, every last one of them.

I had just plain good luck with my wheels. 'Course that buzzard in Texas gave me a start. And that chap in the Chicago Loop who ran into me while I was backing up unnerved me.

The third good thing I've done is write this book. And as Hood Littlefield said, "I hope it helps somebody."

I believe I'll go about getting a little bunch of money together, buy a piece of land, maybe in the Ozarks, throw a few seeds in the ground and get me a couple of swarms.

Awfully glad you came along—and good luck to you.

Perhaps I'll git on down the road now.

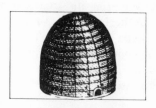

APPENDIX

From the *Washington Post,* May 19, 1974

ARTHRITIS AND BEES
Venom Research Overcoming Old Prejudices
by Patrick Frazier

By MAY OF 1934, 29-year-old Vermont beekeeper Charles Mraz still had acute arthritic pain in his knees from an attack of rheumatic fever the previous January. Just standing up made him wince, and at times he walked like someone three times his age. But it was spring and work had to be done in the apiary.

Mraz had heard the old folk tale about bee stings as a remedy for arthritis, but like most people believed it to be nonsense, especially since he was a beekeeper with arthritis. But, with nothing to lose, he decided to experiment. He caught two bees and made them sting the inside of his knees where the pain was most severe. Two welts raised from the stings but nothing else happened. He soon forgot about it and continued working.

The next morning as he eased out of bed, Mraz suddenly realized that the pain was completely gone. "I said, 'My God, am I imagining that I had arthritis yesterday, or is it my imagination that I haven't got it today?' To this day I cannot believe what happened. That was the start of my interest in BV therapy."

BV stands for bee venom, specifically honeybee venom, the substance injected through the bee's stinger like a hypodermic needle. And BV therapy is the treatment of arthritis with that venom. It's a treatment that for more than a century has had one foot solidly planted in the realm of folk medicine, and the other unsteadily on the ground of established medical practice. But now, from the beginnings of professional research, there are reasons to take bee venom seriously.

Exactly how, where and when bee stings got into the folk pharmacopeia is somewhat of a mystery. There were several classical and medieval remedies calling for the whole honeybee to be used in "prescriptions" that were supposed to cure everything from dysentery to baldness.

A writer on Russian folk medicine claims that bee stings for arthritis have a 300-year history in that country and another says that the oldest German archives indicate it as a cure for gout. Certainly the longest continued use of the venom occurs in homeopathy, a form of medicine that has itself struggled for recognition as a legitimate practice since its inception in the early 1800s.

Within the established 19th Century medical world, Dr. Phillip Terc of Austria was the first extensively to treat arthritics with live bees, giving up to 2,000 stings in a year to some patients. Terc said he became a believer in the healing power of honey-bee stings after an unwanted encounter cured him of his own stubborn muscular rheumatism.

During the 1870s he then "took the risk," he said, "to administer bee venom on people who suffered from rheumatism and even did not shy away from bribing poor people so as to gain experience with it."

Out of hundreds of cases over a 25-year period, he claimed many successes where other treatments of the time had failed.

But he encountered many difficulties, too, not the least of which was ridicule from his colleagues.

There were problems in handling the bees, dealing with allergic reactions in some patients, overcoming their natural fear of stinging insects and postponing treatments over the winter months, when the bees were inactive. And he admitted, "I often tried to apply bee stings in too long neglected cases, too crippled cases or on cases that were already too poor in health." Yet out of his persistence, Terc developed a protocol for treating arthritis that remains the standard used by the few who have kept this tradition alive for a hundred years.

"APIPUNCTURE"

By the turn of the century this treatment gained publicity, with many laymen relating "cure" stories of their own. In the early 1930s, a few foreign doctors and drug companies produced injectable venoms, which were less troublesome and less painful to administer than actual stings.

Before long, bee venom therapy became almost fashionable. European physicians tried it. Lourdes-type bee spas blossomed, suppliers of bees and beekeeping equipment seized the advertising advantage and two U.S. drug companies joined the competition. The treatment was dubbed with various names, one of the catchier ones being "apipuncture."

Then, in 1935, a book appeared entitled simply, "Bee Venom Therapy," giving the most comprehensive study of the subject up to that time. Its author, Hungarian-born Bodog F. Beck, maintained a beehive in his New York office.

Stressing the injectable venoms, Beck enlarged upon Terc's fundamentals and noted that in some cases bee venom aggravated arthritic symptoms temporarily before relieving them. He claimed that many dramatic results were possible with different forms of arthritis and strongly advocated BV therapy, now that the difficulty of being both a doctor and a beekeeper was removed.

In the next few years, several U.S. physicians gave it a try. They experimented with the foreign and domestic injectable venoms on arthritic patients, but their reports showed mixed results. Most felt that bee venom warranted further study but its performance was inconsistent, primarily because of the crude methods in obtaining the venom. And none of these experiments used the strict scientific controls demanded by medical purists. Dr. Beck himself became disappointed with the injectable venoms, though he steadfastly believed in his live bees.

By 1941, Dr. Beck's death, the revival of gold salts as a treatment and the onset of World War II all but killed BV therapy. During this era, most professional encounters with bee venom were limited to a few, and the majority of doctors and scientists, if they knew of it at all, knew it as the folk legend or in time associated it with quackery. For the next 30 years only a handful of Dr. Beck's followers kept their belief in the honeybee's healing power. Among them was the convinced beekeeper, Charles Mraz.

At 69, Mraz is straight and lean, with a ready smile and youthful animation. Despite some heart trouble as a legacy from the rheumatic fever, he's traveled to Mexico, Europe and even Moscow to discuss bees and bee venom. He operates one of New England's largest apiaries and is internationally recognized for his contributions to beekeeping.

Mraz supplied bees to Dr. Beck and eventually learned his methods. He tried unsuccessfully to interest every new doctor in Middlebury in bee stings, so he began giving free treatments to some of his afflicted friends. Mraz has practiced this ex-officio medicine for nearly 40 years on hundreds of arthritics and claims many successes, some as speedy and spectacular as his own.

Ten years ago, Mraz had his "practice" called to the attention of the Vermont medical board by an alarmed doctor whom he had tried to interest in the therapy. But by then, Mraz was pretty well known and respected so little came of it.

"Every doctor in Vermont knows I do this. As a matter of fact, an arthritis specialist with the state of Vermont—one of his patients told him he was going to go and see me—and he said, 'Oh yes, he's cured a lot of my patients.' So, they all know about me."

CORTISONE DEVELOPED

After the war, BV therapy remained more or less an underground affair and, with the development of synthetic cortisone in 1949, most other treatments were swept away. Cortisone was hailed as a "miracle drug" until doctors gradually learned that high and prolonged dosages of it and its sister drugs produce devastating side effects, described by an Arthritis Foundation pamphlet as "something worse than the rheumatoid disease."

Then in 1962, a rather brash book abruptly reopened the bee venom issue. Written by 80-year-old Dr. Joseph Broadman, it was provocatively titled, "Bee Venom. The Natural Curative for Arthritis and Rheumatism." Broadman opened broadside on the medical establishment, the pharmaceutical industry and the government, accusing them of shortsightedness and of suppressing inexpensive bee venom to push artificial, profitable but dangerous steroids. Reporting 40 cases of his own, Broadman extolled the virtues of bee venom, which was still available from Europe in injectable form, and cited the work of several Russians who claimed success with it.

Near the end of his book he modified much of his enthusiasm by saying, "Often I can only arrest pain or give a partial result. I make no fantastic claims." He, too, eventually, became suspicious about the consistency of the injectable venoms.

The Arthritis Foundation's medical department, under Dr. Ronald Lamont-Havers, made some severe criticism and a local foundation chapter's newsletter pictured the book's title page among "quack items." Broadman promptly responded with a $2.5 million libel suit. It turned out, meanwhile, that only half of Broadman's cited cases actually had received BV therapy. The case was settled out of court with a $5,000 award to Broadman and a mild retraction appeared in a subsequent newsletter. But the book still lay open to the same professional criticism of 30 years before: no scientific study with controls.

During the time that the Broadman controversy was stewing, several scattered events involving honeybee venom were taking place.

Its chemical makeup remained virtually unknown until German scientist E. Habermann sorted out most of the ingredients, naming the two prominent ones mellitin and apamin.

In Russia, N.M. Artemov discovered that bee venom acted on the body through the pituitary and adrenal glands, stimulating cortisone output.

In England, researchers found that an enzyme in the venom provided them with a clue for identifying rheumatoid molecules in the fluid that lubricates joints. And allergists were using it in graduated doses to desensitize the less than 5 per cent of the population that is highly allergic to honey-bee stings.

VENOM COLLECTOR

To meet these needs, Allen W. Benton and others at Cornell University developed a device for collecting venom from a number of bees at one time. Independently, Charles Mraz created a similar but improved model from a secondhand description of a Czechoslovakian device. Until then, the methods either were to hold individual bees and make them sting against a surface or to remove the entire venom sac. The problem with this method was that pollen, dust and the bee's body fragments contaminated the venom and, as with the live bee stings on humans, the honeybee didn't survive.

The new device is an electrically charged grid that rests in or near the hive. Thin, synthetic material stretches under this frame, and bees that alight on it get a mild shock that makes them sting through the material, where the venom collects on the underside. The process takes about two hours, and 10,000 bees to produce one gram of pure venom.

As a bonus, the bees' stingers seldom catch in the material, and about 99 per cent survive the process. The bees are not too happy about it, though, and remain furious for several hours. Anyone within 200 yards who is not heavily covered is apt to get severely stung.

In 1962, a retired vice president of General Electric, Glenn

B. Warren, established with his wife and sons a foundation for arthritis research in areas not being funded by other organizations.

Afflicted relentlessly since he was a teenager, having top rheumatologists attend him and undergoing major surgery, Warren continues at 76 to live in the painfully geared-down arthritic world. He has carried a cane for more than 20 years and lost four inches in height from cartilage deterioration. His brother, mother, grandmother, great-grandmother and a son all have suffered the disease. Glenn Warren hopes that his grandchildren can escape the threatening trend.

A friend and amateur beekeeper suggested that he look into the possibility of bee venom as a field for research. Since Warren had experienced virtually every type of arthritis treatment and had educated himself well on the disease, the proposal seemed as feasible as any other.

He ran a computer search of the literature on bee venom and soon met Benton, Broadman, Mraz and several others experienced with it. Warren decided that the treatment had potential, even though he knew it was too late for bee venom to help his own condition substantially.

He was not universally impressed, however, by how the treatments were handled. Some said there were trigger points that had to be stung or injected; others claimed that the venom's action is systemic and can be effectively injected anywhere. Some said BV therapy was sufficient; others said it had to be supplemented.

Unfamiliar with the professional and governmental complexities involved, Warren has spent the last six years trying to overcome the tinge of quackery that bee venom acquired among medical people, the disinterest of drug companies committed to producing synthetic steroids and the rigorous FDA protocol for new drugs.

Already passing FDA's toxicity tests, it is now bogged down in red tape, awaiting tests on human patients. Warren sought and received help from Dr. John Decker, chief of the Arthritis Section of the National Institute of Arthritis, Metabolic and Digestive Diseases (NIAMDD). Decker has helped guide the project through some of the entanglement and suggested a future course for Warren to follow in gaining professional respect for bee venom.

Meanwhile, Warren was already on his own course for bee venom respectability. In San Francisco, Navy biochemist William Shipman came across bee venom literature, looking for a treatment for his daughter's horse, Star, that had developed arthritis and was recommended by a veterinarian to be destroyed.

Shipman prepared his own injectable venom and says, "In a course of weekly injections for six months, Star was cured," and went on to win several gymkana events. Shipman began conducting experiments with bee venom's constituents, studying their physiological effects. Warren learned of his work and financed more of it for the next few years.

Warren next learned of Maj. James Vick, a Walter Reed scientist who is now chief of neurophysiology at Edgewood Arsenal, Md. Vick had been doing work with venoms and Warren arranged for him to get together with Shipman, conduct more experiments with Army and Navy approval and jointly publish them in scientific journals.

Maj. Vick's tests concentrated on recording cortisone output from the adrenal glands of dogs and monkeys. He discovered that bee venom—when injected subcutaneously, as the bee does when it stings—sharply increased cortisone production and maintained it at high levels for one to three days, depending on the dose. Repeat injections sustained above-normal cortisone levels up to 30 days. It's been known since the late 1940s that cortisone relieves arthritic inflammation and the body is better off if it can produce its own cortisone rather than have it induced artificially.

In later tests with arthritic dogs, where injections were spaced farther apart, Vick measured high cortisone output for nearly four months, and the dogs' mobility tripled. These results came from injections equivalent to 70 bee stings for a human—well within tolerance levels. Reflecting on the folk tradition about bee stings and arthritis, Vick, openly optimistic about bee venom, says, "It looks good. Now we've got a scientific basis for the whole thing."

Maj. Vick has been able to confirm the beneficial action of bee venom in a second series of tests on 20 new dogs, 10 of which are control animals. The tests, so far lasting more than 30 days, have reaffirmed the increased cortisone output, and the arthritic dogs' mobility has increased an average of 50 per cent, their cage activity matching that of the non-arthritic animals.

Most enthusiastic about the tests, Warren remarks, "In front of a great many doctors who should know, I made the statement that, so far as I know, there is no other instrumentality in the medical profession that has the ability to stimulate and maintain a high level of cortisone over a long period of time. And I've never been refuted or contradicted." Dr. Decker concurs, saying that this is "so unique as almost to be unbelievable. I'm unaware of any other compound that sustains cortisone at the level Vick has shown in his tests."

Bee venom's biggest challenge came after Warren talked Dr. Gerald Weissmann, professor of medicine at New York University's School of Medicine, and one of the most respected researchers in rheumatology, into testing Mraz' bee venom on the adjuvant arthritic rat model, the standard model by which new treatments are tested. Everyone close to the bee venom work held their breaths at this point, and Dr. Weissmann admits, "I thought it wouldn't work, frankly."

But after the first series of tests, an enthusiastic letter from him to Warren dispelled the doubts. Dr. Weissmann's tests ultimately showed that whole bee venom, more than its individual constituents, did suppress adjuvant arthritis when the rats were injected twice daily from the day the arthritis was induced.

Unlike many other drugs, bee venom prevented the arthritis from appearing after the injections were stopped, and it caused no adverse side effects. Apparently unaware of Dr. Weissmann's work, British researchers also reported recently in Nature magazine that they had discovered an anti-inflammatory element in bee venom they named Peptide 401. In working with the adjuvant arthritic rat, they too observed that arthritis did not develop after injections were stopped.

Offsetting the optimism of Dr. Weissmann's findings was the fact that when the same dose was given 17 days after the arthritis was established at a moderately severe stage, it did not turn back the disease. How then to account for the many dramatic and lasting benefits claimed by bee venom practitioners remains to be settled in human tests.

Nevertheless, Warren asserts, "I am convinced that for arthritis of relatively recent origin—five to 10 years or less—we can demonstrate a simple, inexpensive and largely effective treatment." Looking at Vick's and Dr. Weissmann's work, confirming bee venom's action through the pituitary gland to the adrenals, Warren says, "Now to me, as an amateur, this meant we might have, with bee venom treatment, eliminated one of the major problems associated with either ACTH or cortisone treatment of arthritis."

He refers to the tendency, with prolonged use of artificial steroids, toward atrophy of the body's own adrenal and pituitary glands. With bee venom, "We think we are working through the pituitary and the adrenal and not atrophying either of those. Now that would be all right, possibly, if we act in such a way that we don't atrophy something ahead of the pituitary—hypothalamus or something of that kind. But there has never been any evidence that old beekeepers—and there are millions of them in the world who've had a lot of bee stings —suffer the kinds of diseases that characterize people who have had an excess of either ACTH or cortisone treatment artificially."

Armed with the new scientifically acceptable studies and hoping to get help with successive and more expensive FDA requirements, Warren gathered together Vic, Dr. Weissmann, Mraz and Dr. Decker in February, 1973, to meet with representatives of Abbott Chemical Co., Dr. Charles Sisk from the Arthritis Foundation and the new deputy director of NIAMDD, Dr. Lamont-Havers.

Warren got little response from the Abbott men, but Drs. Sisk and Lamont-Havers pledged help in finding sponsors for clinical trials and offered their institutions' professional expertise in pursuing a program. Considering the controversy of 10 years previous, this represented quite a turnabout for bee venom. Dr. Sisk remarked, "Vick's study particularly is outstanding work on those dogs and I think it demands further trials."

Dr. Sisk is preparing a Phase II bee venom protocol to be followed by whatever clinics conduct Phase II of FDA's requirements for new drugs.

According to Dr. Sisk, the Arthritis Foundation has agreed to set aside funds contributed which are specifically designated for bee venom research.

Because of prior financial commitments, the foundation will be unable to help bee venom research monetarily during Phase II. But if Phase II proves positive, the foundation can give a direct grant for Phase III, or through its cooperating clinics program it can test bee venom on arthritic patients in a national research effort.

Dr. Weissmann thinks that getting a definitive answer to bee venom's potential requires determining the various actions its constituents have on an organism. And each constituent to be tested on a patient would have to pass the entire FDA basic training. Proper research, in his estimation, would entail five good clinical labs spending more than $100,000 each for two years, with patients tested toward the end of these studies.

Dr. Decker is cautious about bee venom's potential, but thinks it warrants investigating, even if it promises to be just another treatment. "It's my view," he explains, "that we, at this juncture, do need carefully designed studies of rheumatoid arthritis treated with bee venom. I would think that a pilot project involving 30 patients for maybe three or four months would be a very important factor in changing the opinions of lots of people, if he (Warren) got a solidly positive result out of such a study."

STANDARDIZED VENOM

Mraz says he now can produce a pure, standardized injectable venom and, so far, the scientists who have used it agree that it's of consistently good quality. Yet in trying to find a doctor, clinic or drug company to carry research further, Warren still finds the folk image a stumbling block.

Allermed Laboratories, Inc., a San Diego pharmaceutical firm, has agreed to put Mraz' bee venom in injectable form to be used for Phase II clinical tests.

Dr. Weissmann observed that in the adjuvant rats' complicated biological response to bee venom, there appeared the possibility that its arthritis suppression may act in another, undetermined fashion aside from the pituitary-adrenal stimulation. It's conceivable then that this other mode of action, once pinned down, may clarify what is attracting the inflammation in the first place, and thereby help in discovering the disease's cause. "It looks awfully promising," Dr. Weissmann says, "but it's in a rudimentary stage."

Shipman and others found that 80 percent or more of mice injected with bee venom survived when exposed to a lethal dose of radiation 24 hours afterward. Other compounds to be effective as radiation protectors have to be administered just prior to irradiation. Here, too, bee venom is operating in an unknown manner, different from all other compounds, and could provide clues to how the body protects itself.

Hopes are that it may aid in radiation treatment for cancer, if it doesn't protect cancerous cells as well as healthy ones. Lack of funds and facilities halted Shipman's and a coworker's experiments that hinted bee venom may have a positive place in leukemia research.

In work on isolated dog and monkey hearts, Maj. Vick and Shipman discovered a new BV constituent they named cardiopep, which has a pronounced stimulating and stabilizing effect, lasting much longer than other known drugs. This may offer hope to those who suffer from congestive heart failure.

"You know that when you get this damnable disease, your

life span is probably about five years, even with the best drugs," according to Vick. "If cardiopep works as well as it appears to work and is as non-toxic now as Bill thinks it is, then we've got something that may double or even triple that life span."

"We now have it completely purified and isolated and we've tested it," Vick says.

One remarkable experiment concerns a chimpanzee that was in the throes of death from a lethal shock. Respiration had ceased and the heart was undergoing a faint fibrillation when Vick injected cardiopep. The chimp's heart and pulse rate began to stabilize, and after another injection two hours later, the chimpanzee returned to normal and stayed healthy.

Bee venom fans are not surprised by these side effects. They claim to have observed many improvements in maladies other than arthritis.

Dr. Terc, for instance, noticed a hundred years ago that two of his patients' heart irregularities ceased after bee sting treatment.

Ironically, it's been claims like these that convinced most scientists that bee venom was one of those untrustworthy folk panaceas. But scientific preliminaries have so far confirmed much of what honeybee advocates maintained all along. Warren and Mraz have succeeded in focusing attention on an exciting "new drug," but getting things farther requires more people who will listen and help.

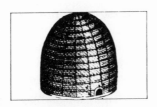

BIBLIOGRAPHY

PERIODICALS

Ainlay, G.W. "The Use of Bee Venom in the Treatment of Arthritis and Neuritis." *Nebraska Medical Journal* 24:298–303 (1939).

Artemov, N.M. "The Biological Bases of the Therapeutic Use of Bee Venom." Department of Physiology, Faculty of Medicine, National University of Gorki, USSR (1959).

Bonimond, J.P. "Perspectives sur l'action du venin d'abeille." *Revue français d'apiculture* (Nov. 1976).

Broadman, Joseph. "Rheumatism and Its Treatment by the General Practitioner." *General Practice* 5:11, 12, 54, 58 (1958).

_____. "A Review of the Foreign Literature on Bee Venom for the Treatment of All Types of Rheumatism." *General Practice* 8:13, 26, 28, 29 (1958).

Cavanagh, Denis, Beazley, John, and Ostapowicz, Frank. "Radical Operation for Carcinoma of the Vulva: A New Approach to Wound Healing." *Journal of Obstetrics and Gynaecology of the British Commonwealth* 77:1037–1040 (1970).

Cho, Young T. "Studies on Royal Jelly and Abnormal Cholesterol and Triglycerides." *American Bee Journal* 1:36–38 (1977).

Church, Julia. "Honey as a Source of the Anti-Stiffness Factor." *Federation Proceedings* (March 1954).

Crane, Eva. "Honey: Past, Present and Future." *American Bee Journal* 3:142 (1977).

Edwards, Thyra. "Bee Stings Cured My Arthritis." *Pageant Magazine* (Mar. 1953).

Foundation for Nutrition and Stress *Research Bulletin,* March 1969.

Frazier, Patrick. "Arthritis and Bees." *Washington Post,* May 19, 1974, pp. c1, c5.

Guyton, F.E. "Bee Sting Therapy for Arthritis and Neuritis." *Journal of Economic Entomology* 40(4):469 (1947).

Haydak, Mykola H. "Bee Venom." *Iowa State Apiarist* (1951).

Hayes, Bernie. "Propolis and the Balm-of-Gilead." *American Bee Journal* 3:148–149 (1977).

Kemp, F. Roy. "Athletes Use Pollen for Performance." *Let's Live* (July 1976).

Kononenko, I.F. "Bee Venom Preparation Mellissin as a Remedy and Disease Preventing Agent." Paper delivered at XVII International Congress of Apiculture, Rome, 1958.

Kroner, J., Lintz, R., Tyndall, M., Anderson, L., and Nichols, E. "The Treatment of Rheumatoid Arthritis with an Injectable Form of Bee Venom." *Annals of Internal Medicine* 2(7):1077–1088 (1938).

Lorenzetti, G.J., Fortenberry, B., and Busby, E. "Influence of Bee Venom in the Adjuvant-Induced Arthritic Rat Model." *Research Communications in Chemical Pathology and Pharmacology* 4(2): (Sept. 1972).

Montagny, Hubert Stern. "Bee Venom Therapy." *Gleanings in Bee Culture* 1:42 (1943).

Montgomery, Paul L. "Bee Pollen: Wonder Drug or Humbug?" *New York Times,* Feb. 6, 1977, Sec. 5, pp. 1, 7.

Mraz, Charles. "Bee Venom Therapy." *American Bee Journal* 4:260 (1977).

––––––. "The 2nd International Apitherapy Congress." *American Bee Journal* 2:86, 87 (1977).

New York Center Research Institute, Inc., *Annual Report*

Nichols, E.E. "Rheumatoid Arthritis Treatment with the Sting of the Honey Bee." *New York State Medical Journal* 38:1218 (1938).

Root, E.R. "The Remedial Value of Stings." *Gleanings in Bee Culture* 1:16–20; 2:84–87 (1935).

_____. "Bee Venom." *Gleanings in Bee Culture* 8:492–495 (1938).

Ryan, Don. "Dr. Carey's Bees Vanquish Arthritis." *American Bee Journal* 1:11, 13 (1977).

Saine, Joseph. Lecture delivered at the Eighth Annual Meeting of Eastern Apicultural Society, University of Vermont, Burlington, August 24, 1962.

_____. "Is Bee Venom a Panacea in the Treatment of Arthritis?" Paper presented at International Symposium on Apitherapy, Bucharest, 1965.

_____. Lecture to the International Academy of Preventive Medicine, Kansas City, Sept. 12, 1976.

Schweisheimer, W. "Cancer and Beekeeping." *Gleanings in Bee Culture* 9:360, 561 (1967).

Vick, James A. "Therapeutic Applications of Bee Venom and Its Components in the Dog." *American Bee Journal* 11:414–416 (1972).

Vick, James A., Warren, Glenn B., and Brooks, Robert. "The Effect of Treatment with Whole Bee Venom on Daily Cage Activity and Plasma Cortisol Levels in the Arthritic Dog." *American Bee Journal* 2:52, 53, 58 (1975).

Waldt, Felix S., Mathers, H., and Damrau, Frederic. "Standardized Bee Venom (SBV) Therapy of Arthritis." *Industrial Medicine and Surgery* 12:1045–1049 (1966).

Weissmann, G., et al. "Effect of Bee Venom on Experimental Arthritis." *Annals of the Rheumatic Diseases* 32:466–470 (1973).

Wells, F.B. "Hive Product Uses—Royal Jelly." *American Bee Journal* 12:560, 561, 565 (1976).

_____. "Hive Product Uses—Venom." *American Bee Journal* 1:10, 12, 22 (1977).

Yunginger, John W. "Recent Diagnostic and Therapeutic Advances in Stinging Insect Allergy." *American Bee Journal* 115 (8):308–309 ( ).

BOOKS

Beck, Bodog. *Bee Venom Therapy.* New York: Appleton, 1935.

_____. *Honey and Health.* New York: Robert McBride, 1938.

Binding, George J. *About Pollen.* London: Thorson, 1971.

Broadman, Joseph. *Bee Venom: The Natural Curative for Arthritis and Rheumatism.* New York: Putnam, 1962.

Dufty, William. *Sugar Blues.* New York: Warner Books, 1976.

Harnaj, Eng, et al. *Apimondia Scientific Bulletin.* Bucharest: Apimondia, 1972.

———. *The Hive Products, Food, Health and Beauty.* Madrid: International Symposium on Apitherapy, 1974.

———. *Apitherapy Today.* Bucharest: Apimondia, 1976.

Ioyrish, Naum. *Curative Properties of Honey and Bee Venom.* Moscow: Foreign Languages Publishing House, 1959.

———. *Bees and People.* Moscow: MIR, 1974.

Jarvis, D.C. *Arthritis and Folk Medicine.* Greenwich: Fawcett, 1960.

———. *Folk Medicine.* London: Pan Books, 1975.

McCormick, Marjorie. *The Golden Pollen.* Yakima: Yakima Binding & Printing, 1960.

Murat, Felix. *Bee Pollen: Miracle Food.* Miami: Murat, 1976.

Nichols, Joe D. *Please, Doctor, Do Something!* Old Greenwich: Devin-Adair, 1975.

Owens, Julia. *Doctors Without Shame.* Kent: Julia Owens Publications, 1965.

Perlman, Dorothy. *The Magic of Honey.* New York: Hearst, 1974.

Root, A.I. *ABC & XYZ of Bee Culture.* Medina: Root, 1975.

Smith, Adam. *Powers of Mind.* New York: Ballantine Books, 1976.

von Frisch, Karl. *The Dancing Bees.* New York: Harcourt, 1953.

Wallace, Irving, and Wallechinsky, David. *People's Almanac.* Garden City, N.Y.: Doubleday, 1975.